Clowns and Jokers Can Heal Us

Comedy and Medicine

D0872512

Perspectives in Medical Humanities

Perspectives in Medical Humanities publishes scholarship produced or reviewed under the auspices of the University of California Medical Humanities Consortium, a multi-campus collaborative of faculty, students and trainees in the humanities, medicine, and health sciences. Our series invites scholars from the humanities and health care professions to share narratives and analysis on health, healing, and the contexts of our beliefs and practices that impact biomedical inquiry.

General Editor

Brian Dolan, PhD, Professor of Social Medicine and Medical Humanities, University of California, San Francisco (UCSF)

Forthcoming Titles

The Remarkables: Endocrine Abnormalities in Art
By Carol Clark and Orlo Clark (Autumn 2011)

Paths to Innovation: Discovering Recombinant DNA, Oncogenes, and Prions in One Medical School, Over One Decade
By Henry Bourne (Fall, 2011)

Health Citizenship: Essays in Social Medicine and Biomedical Politics
By Dorothy Porter (Fall, 2011)

Darwin and the Emotions: Mind, Medicine, and the Arts
Edited by Angelique Richardson and Brian Dolan (Summer, 2012)

www.medicalhumanities.ucsf.edu

brian.dolan@ucsf.edu

This series is made possible by the generous support of the Dean of the School of Medicine at UCSF, the Center for Humanities and Health Sciences at UCSF, and a Multi-Campus Research Program grant from the University of California Office of the President.

For Rebecca and Gustavo

Clowns and Jokers Can Heal Us

Comedy and Medicine

Albert Howard Carter III

First published in 2011

by UC Medical Humanities Consortium and distributed by UC Press.

BERKELEY — LOS ANGELES — LONDON

© 2011

University of California

Medical Humanities Consortium

3333 California Street, Suite 485

San Francisco, CA 94143-0850

Cover Art by Ian MacNeil

Library of Congress Control Number: 2011932614

ISBN 978-0-9834639-1-7

Printed in USA

Contents

Figures

Acknowledgments

M ANY KIND PEOPLE have sent me or told me jokes and given me other examples; many thanks to them all: Avise Nissen, Carolyn and Lloyd Horton, Susan and T. J. Gill, Steve Stambaugh, Dana Durst Lawrence, Julie Empric, George Meese, James G. Crane, J. Thomas West, Peter Meinke, Harry Ellis, Robert Detweiler, Beth and Vaughn Morrison, Mary Ann Willis, Robert Hetzel, John and Margaret Scanlan, Rich and Mimi Rice, P. Martha Graham, Alice and Bill Fadden, Chad Wilson, Tom and Marian Price, Allan Friedman, Jane Arbuckle Petro, David Fleischer, Bill Nesmith, Chris Mazzaro, George Gopen, Brad Davis, and David Howell.

My thanks to those who have encouraged this project over the years: the late Joanne Trautmann Banks, also Jay Baruch, James F. Childress, Rebecca Garden, Laurence B. McCullough, Lois Nixon, Warren Reich, Mahala Yates Stripling, David Watts, and Delese Wear. I thank also Felice Aull, Rita Charon, Jack Coulehan, Ann Hudson Jones, Therese Jones, Kathryn Montgomery, and Audrey Shafer for their inspiring work in the medical humanities field.

Presentations of some of this material include national meetings of the Society for Values in Higher Education, both in the Popular Culture morning groups and as a Fellows Memorial lecture (San Diego, 2001), the Faculty Forum of the Social Medicine Department, School of Medicine, University of North Carolina-Chapel Hill, and the Food for Thought program at Eckerd College.

For superb help with research and copy editing, I thank Susan Yael Siegel; for bibliographical matters, Chris Mazzaro; for computer assistance, Ron Evans, and for brainstorming, Chris Osmond. For assistance with illustrations, I thank Eddie Staples of the Office of Information Systems, UNC School of Medicine. For acquiring and guiding this study, my warm thanks go to Brian Dolan, editor, Perspectives in Medical Humanities.

I provide massage for cancer patients through the Patient and Family Resource Center on the North Carolina Cancer Hospital; I thank my coworkers Tina Shaban, Pamela Baker, and Beth Fogel. Our center is part of the Comprehensive Cancer Support Program, and I thank Donald L. Rosenstein, the director. This program is part of Lineberger Comprehensive Cancer Center at UNC-Chapel Hill. I thank the nurses I work with in the Bone Marrow Transplant Unit there: Jody Allen, Murial "Missy" Beckwith, Josh Bradley, Amy Byington, Tiffany Carr, Kelly Colvin, Karah Daniel, Ashley Farmer, Joe Kleinman, Amy Leiser, Angela Spruill, and Gayl Talbert, also Recreational Therapists Kelly Kivette and Michelle Barr.

I also thank the nurses in the Outpatient Infusion Center: Mala Ananthan, Stacey Anderegg, Elizabeth Bell, Patricia Decator, Amy De Pue, Michelle Gifford, Jan Gremillion, Sue Haney, Tish Harris, Elizabeth Kizer, Clare Kneis, Lori Kramer, Stacey Jones, Linda McElveen, Patti Morfeld, Ann Nowrouzzadeh, Jerome Schiro, Beth Springthorpe, and Julie White. Also oncology patient coordinator Jennifer Byrd.

I also thank pharmacist Chris Walko, oncology chaplain Patricia Cadle, and nurse and fellow massage therapist Chris Clark.

Physicians who have kept me going include Richard Oldenski, Andrew Peterson, Eugene Orringer, Carolyn Sidor, Arthur Axelbank, and Niall Buckley. I thank them all.

Writing is often lonely work, and friends are especially important. I thank Diana Grove, Bruce and Carol Hewitt, Colleen Adomaitis, George and Karen Meese, Tom and Marian Price, Bill and Diane Savage, Jane Rectanwald and Fran Weigand, Dixie McLaughlin, and Nikole Weir. Also Jerry and Betty Eidenier, Albert and Janet Rabil, Carl and Janet Edwards, Ken Jens and Sandy Milroy Jens, Judy and Glenn Morris, Mark and Allison Davidson, Katie Ricks and Paula Gibbs, Charlie and Nancy Zimmerli, Janet Boudreau, and Tom and Nancy Trueblood.

I thank family members Janet and Ian MacNeil, Marilyn and David Keeser, Bette and Sky Weeks, Martin and Erin Stuart. Also Cliff and Sheri Carter, Jimmy and Delores Carter, Ronald and Monica Carter, Scott and Huong Carter. Also Alex Carter Gudger and Elizabeth Frances Carter. I thank my late parents Howard and Marjorie Carter, and my late sister Avise Elizabeth Nisssen. I thank my daughter Rebecca Alice-Carter Rincon and her husband Gustavo and my wife Nancy Corson Carter.

I thank successive chairs of Social Medicine, School of Medicine, UNC-Chapel Hill: Desmond K. Runyan, Alan W. Cross, and Gail E. Henderson.

—AHC

Introduction

THE OVER-ARCHING PURPOSE of comedy—whether a funny movie, a practical joke, a Shakespearean comedy, a pun, or a joke about doctors—is to affirm energy and freedom. The community involved may be as small as two people exchanging jokes, a large crowd in a theater, or world-wide users of the Internet. The sharing involves conventions in narrative and rituals of telling, hearing, and laughing. Comedy is a strange enterprise: some of its features are rational, but many are irrational. It has conventions that are highly predictable but also elements of surprise and absurdity. It can range from gentle play with language to vicious, attacking humor, from a skillful parody to a Hollywood movie. In many, many forms, comedy appears to be universal, around the world and throughout all human time. In many cases, it is a positive resource, bonding people together, although in some cases, it may be divisive and hurtful. Especially in cases where people are sick, comedy should be used carefully.

Comedy works best when there are shared values. When arriving for a comic play, a comedian's show, or a circus, an audience knows what to expect. When a group of friends tell jokes, they know what kinds of humor are acceptable. When there are social differences, however, comedy may not work or, indeed, it may be harmful; a joke that bosses tell about a workplace may not be funny to the workers. In the medical world there are marked differences in status and power within the medical personnel, from attending physicians down to nurses, techs, and support staff. In hospitals and clinics, there is another and enormous difference between the caregivers—who are at work practicing their craft and earning money and who are, typically, healthy—and the patients, whose lives have been disrupted and who are anxious, afraid, perhaps even terrified. Medical caregivers sometimes use gentle humor with patients to cheer them up, but, among themselves, they use humor which can be wild, even harsh.

If we visit someone in the hospital, crossing from the world of the well to the world of the sick, we commonly seek to *cheer up* the patient, using humor (typically gentle) in order to include the patient back into the world of the well (and, also, to maintain ourselves while we are there). Patients are usually grateful to be reintegrated

medicine has created
a hierarchy that dieifize
MD

into normal society, if only symbolically and temporarily, and joking is one efficient means to accomplish that.

Well people in the world of the well often enjoy jokes about sick people as fictional characters who don't feel pain; such humor allow us to maintain a separation from that other, frightening world, while ritually acknowledging that it does, nonetheless, exist. Some of these jokes can be extreme, well beyond the norms of polite society.

Even sick people sometimes share humor among themselves to affirm that they still embody aspects of wellness, imagination, and freedom. As a cancer patient, I recall the first time I saw—and laughed at—another patient cheerfully wearing a button that read "CANCER SUCKS."

Some comedy is scripted, for example in plays, movies, and books. These contributions by professional writers are important in their own right—and I'll allude to some—but in this book I'm more interested in (1) the comedy that emerges in medical settings and (2) comedy about medicine that we find in jokes shared in the oral tradition, told and retold with variations by many or even all of us. With the advent of email, Google, and humor websites, the cyber realm now sends jokes with lightning speed to anywhere in the world, widely expanding the reach of the oral tradition, although not necessarily the nature of jokes. According to Holt, some theorists believe that there are no new jokes, only retold and evolving ones.[1] I've been collecting jokes about medical topics for some 25 years; they are from many sources, including conversation around the copy machine, email from relatives, friends, and colleagues who knew of my strange project, and, more lately, the Internet, where sites list hundreds and hundreds of jokes. Clearly this is a commonplace activity. What does it mean? What purposes do jokes serve? How do they work? Do they contribute to our mental health? In what senses may we say that they heal us?

Jokes on the page, on our computer screens, or even in the air between two people are abstract in the sense that they are stories without direct connection to actual events. Neither history nor journalism, jokes are esthetic fictions that we enjoy hearing and telling; they are "short, short stories," with their own esthetic structures, such as character types, quickly climactic plots, and punch lines. Jokes are entertainments that create an imaginative world, and when we visit this world we enter a consciousness that literary critics have called the Green World, an ideal place of health, fertility, abundance, and joy.

When there is no audience present, there is a further abstraction: gone are the shared values of a comic community, gone are the teller's inflections, gestures, facial expressions, and variations in voice, all of which help communicate the speaker's intentions.

So I'll say it straight out here: my intent is to define and describe comedy in all its resources in order to understand how it can contribute to healing sick people and supporting the health of well people, and, also, to suggest ways it should be limited to avoid harm. I'll illustrate my claims with real-life examples from hospitals and clinics as well as with jokes I have collected over the years. Obviously, I have no sense of which examples will be enjoyed by which readers, so I urge them to pick the ones they do like (and ignore unacceptable ones) in order to consider the points I seek to make.

We may call the real-life examples "emergent," happening in the moment, such as a series of puns or other witticisms that people say extemporaneously. Emergent humor in the hospital is akin to improv comedy, made up on the spot. I've been a volunteer in hospitals for some twenty years and a massage therapist in a hospital for another five, encountering humor of all sorts, from the gentle to the outrageous. When I was a volunteer in the Emergency Room, there was a wide variety, from kind humor with patients to dramatic, even crazy humor among the caregivers. Through the ER doors came ample evidence that the world can be a place of chaos and suffering, to which ER nurses and doctors had to respond quickly and efficiently, at any hour of the day or night. Sometimes these workers attempted to protect, maintain, and heal themselves through comic visits to the Green World, as we'll see in Chapters Three and Eleven.

One of the purposes of this book is to make connections between the somewhat abstract world of jokes as they are written or told and the lived reality of patients and caregivers in the clinic and hospital. I will show that the purposes of comedy are the same in both realms.

COMEDY, HUMOR, AND MEDICINE

What is the relation of comedy and humor? The terms overlap, of course, but my emphasis for "humor" will be the *quality* that makes something—a joke, a pun, an image—funny, something that makes us smile, chuckle, or laugh out loud. The term "comedy" emphasizes the *activities* of being funny in social ways. Whether we're in a small or a large group, we participate in rituals of laughter and affirmation that nourish our identities as social persons and our relationships to others. Comedy is transactional; someone tells a joke, other people laugh. Further, comic narratives typically emphasize stories of restoration of a society, as in the ending of the Shakespearean comedy, such as *Much Ado about Nothing*, when two marriages bring men and women together and make possible the creation of children, effectively the next generation assuring that society will continue. Some of the values ritually affirmed on stage (and for the audience) include the health of spouses, sexual pleasure and procreation, social coherence and continuity, as well as, of course, love and happiness. Because comic narratives end by resolving conflicts, they provide hope that it is possible to pass from chaos into a new normalcy.

In a doctor's office or a hospital, we welcome humor that makes us feel that we are still part of the larger, healthy human family, even though we may be physically unwell. Such humor holds us in the world of the well, even though we are sick. At a deeper level, we yearn for an implicit story that sketches our health, our current unhealthy state, and our future (soon, we hope) health. In myth studies, the Night Sea Journey is a primal story of normalcy, descent into danger, and ascent back to normalcy and health, for example the story of Jonah and the Whale, while other versions, such as the story of Job, use a psychological fall and rise instead of a spatial journey. Dante called his great poem a *commedia*, because it was a story with a happy ending in Paradise after the arduous journey through the Inferno and Purgatory. In religious terms, a comedic character is *redeemed*, bought back from separation, even exile. For persons who believe in heaven, dying and entering an eternal life is the ultimate comic story.

Comedy is intensely social. It is also pleasurable, something we choose to participate in because we like it. Comedy reminds us of social ideals that are important to us, such as health, caring, love, sexual pleasure, and, in general, joy. And, yes, there are times when comedy is not appropriate; it is not a cure-all, and there are times when it doesn't work or can even be harmful.

Comedy and medicine. What can the two terms share besides the gratuitous syllable "med"? Medicine is, of course, involved with healing, that is, bringing sick or injured people from suffering and loss of function back to the best health possible, and modern medicine does many wonderful things, things that earlier ages would deem miraculous. Palliative medicine—a recent development—helps people at the end of life to another kind of healing. At the same time, however, pressures of time, economics, technology, and more have made the delivery of some, even much, medical care impersonal, so that a patient may feel dehumanized, even to the status of a lab rat. The purpose of this book is to emphasize human caring through comedy that (1) enhances medical care, whether in clinic, hospital, rehab facility, nursing home, or a bedroom at home and that (2) helps to keep us healthy, whether we are caregivers or ordinary, well people.

At a deep level, comedy can affirm life, caring, and love.

A word about the term "medicine," a term that might, strictly speaking, apply to drugs and surgery, and not the wider meaning for care of sick bodies in general. Decades ago Ivan Illich complained that *medicalizing* our health was misguided, because it collapsed all aspects of healthcare into the idea that the interventions of hospitals, doctors, and drugs are the only approach to staying well.[2] When our bodies are routinely *medicalized*, we have a limited way of perceiving them, often losing some, much, or even all of our control. We may even give up personal and social responsibility for understanding health and caring for it. Instead, I would prefer the terms "healthcare" or "health maintenance," because they suggest that taking care of our bodies and minds is an ongoing process, even when we are well, and not just when we become sick or have an injury. Although somewhat paradoxical, the phrase "preventive medicine" expands the notion that medicine can support and extend health, and it is this larger sense that is important to me in writing about comedy, because I see comedy as a kind of preventive medicine or health maintenance strategy as well as an adjunct to medical care of patients. Of course, the terms "medicine" and "medical" are now ubiquitous, so I must use them here, but I want to include their larger meanings of promoting the health of body and mind as well as the interventive medicine we commonly know. The phrase "literature and medicine" now indicates a relatively new professional subfield, with its own journal (with that exact name), which is a part of the larger field of "medical humanities," a phrase that now has currency despite the problems, again, of contemporary medicine's limitations. (I would prefer "healthcare humanities.") When I refer to medical topics, I don't mean only doctors, surgery, and drugs—as important as they are—but the wider sense of health and healthcare that includes, maintains, and heals both the well and the sick.

How I Came To This Project

I've been fascinated by jokes, puns, comedy, humor, and games for a long time. While I was growing up, my family played with all of these, delighting in their novelty, variety, and surprise. In college and graduate school, I studied comedy with pleasure, but also with the nagging sense that I wasn't getting the full story, because literary studies in the days of the New Criticism paid no attention to the social behaviors that made comedy powerful. I might be reading Molière in class, but no professor made links to the jokes that students routinely shared outside of class or the comic movies or TV shows we watched. I sensed that comedy was a living dynamic central to life itself, but I found no texts that explained that for me. The Ivory Tower made comedy a set of abstractions, removed from how people actually lived.

During the second half of my career as a literature professor, I became involved with this new subfield of literature and medicine. This hybrid focus for research and writing led me to many unusual places: burn units, anatomy labs, cardiology units—all of which I have written about.[3] These were places of dramatic reality and concrete specificity, inhabited by real people, both patients and caregivers. They were also places where humor played a vital role. After training as an E.M.T., I was a pastoral care volunteer in an urban Emergency Room/Trauma Center for a dozen years. Outsiders would sometimes ask me, "I've heard that the ER has a weird sense of humor; is this true?" as if that humor were abnormal, a deviant humor that was well beyond the pale. Perhaps no one should want to go to an ER because people who worked there were clearly unhealthy! During my time in the ER, I observed humor of many sorts, much of it like humor in other places, but also some humor that was, by ordinary social standards, extreme. ER humor—like humor in other high-stress places in the hospital such as in ICUs, the burn unit, or operating rooms—was a mixture of moods and topics, all of them with the purpose of maintaining the social bonds of the working groups involved. Such dynamics enlivened the widely watched movie and TV series *M*A*S*H*, which were based on Richard Hooker's novel *Mash* (1968).[4] Indeed, writing about comedy and medicine has much more been the purview of popular culture media and fiction writers, for example Samuel Shem's perennial classic *House of God* (1978),[5] than a topic for theorists. Medical humanists are generally intelligent, witty, even hilarious people, but their conference presentations and publications tend to focus on serious matters, of which there have been plenty: Baby Fae, "Debbie," Dax Cowart, Terri Schiavo, inequalities in care, implications for new technologies, disability studies, the US healthcare "system," and so on.

The ER was, of course, a portal to the rest of the hospital. I'd often help take patients upstairs, either in a wheelchair to OB or on a gurney to a room or to an ICU. Sometimes I'd visit a patient a week later to see how he or she was doing. My volunteer's jacket could get me into most places of the hospital, including the OR suite and the morgue, and I was later a volunteer in the cardiac service, a cancer ward, and Rehab. I found humor and comedy in all of these places, except the morgue, isolated in the basement behind a locked, unlabeled door.

JOKERS, CLOWNS, NORMAN COUSINS, PATCH ADAMS

Jokers are of many sorts, from gentle punsters to outrageous stand-up comics. We tell jokes because they entertain us, change our mood, and allow for sharing between teller and listener, thus creating social bonds. We tell jokes about medical topics because we need ways to deal with our fears about illness, pain, debility, dependence, and death. The other side of a specific fear, for example the fear of aging, is an affirmation of the values that are at risk: vitality, active minds, sexuality, freedom, and the like. Much humor affirms values that are central to us. Even satiric or sarcastic humor affirms positive values when it attacks HMOs, greedy doctors, bossy nurses, or the indignities of hospitalization, such as loss of privacy, institutional food, and hospital gowns.

A subset of jokers, clowns are typically conventional figures immediately recognizable by costume and makeup. Whether at a circus, a birthday party, or a hospital, clowns bring familiarity and comfort because they have the well defined role of entertaining us in friendly, non-threatening ways. But there are other important qualities. Because clowns fit in tiny cars, have mock fights but never get hurt, and fall down only to rise up unharmed, clowns embody a supernatural vitality and physical invulnerability. Clowns may seem ordinary—normal people in costumes—but they exemplify extraordinary abilities to overcome physical laws of space as well as ordinary human limits, even mortality. As we shall see, there are also clown-like figures not in costume and makeup, persons who play similar roles of entertaining and demonstrating the power of comic vitality.

We have, then, several kinds of jokers and clowns. Well people tell jokes in a relaxed atmosphere. Well healthcare workers use gentle humor with patients but also ironic humor among themselves in stressful settings such as a burn unit or an emergency department. Sick patients sometimes tell jokes to each other; I've seen burn units where patients wore buttons that read CRISPY CRITTER. And well people sometimes joke with sick patients, for example, a hospital clown visiting patients' rooms.

In recent decades, two figures—one a patient, the other a doctor—have attracted attention because they have combined the notions of comedy and health. One is Norman Cousins, whose book *Anatomy of an Illness as Perceived by the Patient: Reflections on Healing and Regeneration* (1979) described how he laughed himself well by watching Marx Brothers movies.[6] I read this book when it came out and was fascinated by the possibility. Was there, indeed, truth to the common phrase "laughter is the best medicine"? Should we be tempted to do away with doctors who are all too serious and also hospitals that are ugly, impersonal, and, basically, inhospitable? Are there ways that comedy can overcome some of these obstacles? While the book drew much popular attention, comedy did not, of course, replace medicine.

Patch Adams, a doctor and a clown, gained much publicity through the Robin Williams movie "Patch Adams" (1989), but his work at the Gesundheit Institute in West Virginia has been ongoing since 1971. He has published two books, *Gesundheit!*

(1998) and *House Calls: How We Can Heal the World One Visit at a Time* (1998).[7] I've heard Patch speak. He was wearing strange, mismatched clothes and a necktie that looked like a trout. "These are my working clothes," he said. "I'm a clown." According to his 2008 website, "Dr. Patch Adams and members of the Gesundheit Institute have lectured at medical and nursing schools in over 65 countries and on five continents, reaching approximately 150,000 attendees per year. Over 1,300 people per year participate in Gesundheit's medical student electives, volunteer programs, alternative spring breaks, healthcare system design intensives, humanitarian clown trips, and health justice gatherings." A leader in humanizing the delivery of healthcare across the globe, Patch uses clowning and humor in general to transform medicine.

While these two have been the most visible figures of comedy and medicine, thousands of doctors, nurses, and other caregivers share humor with patients every day, helping patients feel that they are still part of the human community, even when they are sick. This important activity is, and should be, a central part of the delivery of medical care.

LAUGHTER, THEORY, BIOETHICS

It's been said that explaining something funny is neither possible nor appropriate, in the sense that, once explained, it can no longer be funny. There's some truth to that: we laugh when we make immediate, unconscious connections within the right kind of mood. If we try to explain a funny moment later, our listeners may not "get it," and we often end up with, "Well, I guess you had to have been there." But humor is not a will-o'-the-wisp never to be captured, and theorists of many sorts have made interesting and helpful contributions. One approach is the physiological, explaining dynamics of laughter (see Sakuragi et al.),[8] while another is evolutionary, speculating that the deep origins of laughter were sources of human bonding (Gervais and Wilson).[9] Another more clearly medical approach is from nursing, which often stresses the affective dimensions of patient care. A large number of articles show psychological and physiological links between health and comedy, humor, and laughter; these include MRI studies, improved immune function, pain reduction, stress reduction, lowering blood pressure, and so on. C. Hassad and Hélène Patenaude have reviewed much of this research.[10] Bennett and Lengacher specifically write that humor helps to relieve stress, can improve mental health, and supports quality of life.[11] I imagine (and hope) that such studies will continue and will eventually coalesce to show definitively that comedy provides curative effects and health benefits.

Writers about literature and medicine tend to treat narrative as serious and utilitarian, ideally part of delivery of proper health care, with applications for the training of physicians, developing competencies, and bioethical implications. Anne Hudson Jones has provided an excellent overview, stressing connections with medical ethics.[12] Similarly, Howard Brody's essay "My Story Is Broken; Can You Help Me Fix It" emphasizes the joint construction of narrative by physician and patient to deal with a patient's illness.[13] Brody also mentions "symbolical healing" of careful listening which helps to set "a tone of care and compassion" (p. 80) and the need for "reattachment to the human community from which the patient, through illness, has been cut off" (p. 86); I believe that appropriate humor can serve these two therapeutic aims.

Some of the most important contributions on literature and medicine tend to do little or nothing with comedy, emphasizing instead medical knowledge, clinical judgment, medical training, or delivery of medicine. As helpful as they are in other ways, Anne Hunsaker Hawkins' *Reconstructing Illness: Studies in Pathography*, Kathryn Montgomery Hunter's *Doctors' Stories*, her *How Doctors Think*, and Rita Charon's *Narrative Medicine* do not advance our understanding of comedy and medicine. I believe my case for comedy as an adjunct to medicine supplements the arguments of both Hunter and Charon. I think of Paul Horton's title and subtitle, *Solace: The Missing Dimension in Psychiatry*; comedy has similarly been missing in serious writing about medicine.[14] I hope this study will help fill that gap.

In "Narrative-Based Medicine: Potential, Pitfalls, and Practice," Kalitzkus and Matthiessen discuss patient stories, physicians' stories, narratives about physician-patient encounters, and "grand stories" or metanarratives, without any emphasis on comedy.[15] My discussion will include most of these, with an emphasis on the metanarratives of comic plots, such as stories of reintegration and the Night Sea Journey. Their article states that narrative-based medicine arose to counteract shortcomings of evidence-based medicine, but concludes, sensibly enough, that the latter is always necessary and the former can often be helpful. Jeffrey P. Bishop, on the other hand, sees the same unfortunate philosophical underpinnings of instrumental thinking beneath standard medicine and medical humanities, including narrative medicine, concluding with his judgment of *a plague on both your houses*.[16] I think instrumentality can be a very good thing in the medical realm and that comedy can be well used for a purpose of making a patient feel at ease, but also for no utilitarian purpose at all, simply (and powerfully) as an act that affirms existential freedom.

My view is that standard medicine should routinely use any possible benefits from the humanities to nourish and support caregivers, patients, and the public at large, and I'll argue specifically for comedy in various forms as an adjunct to medical care.

My approach owes much to my training in comparative literature, a discipline that considers continuities across the literary arts, even unusual and disparate kinds. I draw on a mixture of classic literary theory, my own clinical observation and interpretation, and my personal experience as a patient. One more person in the oral tradition (and not a folklorist), I have retold many of the jokes and combined others, especially when I've heard or read several versions.

Aims Of This Book

Summing up our discussion so far and organizing it, I have four aims for this study.

First, I will present and describe a wide range of comedy in order to chart the many varieties and uses of humor that deals with sickness and injury, medical treatments, even death. I'll provide vignettes from hospitals and clinics, describing instances I have seen over some twenty-eight years as an observer in hospitals and clinics, as a volunteer, as a massage therapist in clinical settings, and as a patient. I'll also present jokes that I have collected, from friends, from hospital personnel, and from the Internet, where there are now hundreds readily available. While the basic mission of hospitals is, of course, serious, the humor found there is more pervasive and more important than we ordinarily assume.

Second, I'll analyze the elements of humor, using literary concepts to illuminate the structures of jokes and their primal appeals. Some aspects of humor are conventional and highly predictable, even rational, but much of its power comes from irrational elements, including surprise, fantasy, the breaking of taboos about illness, death, and sex, and our needs for various rituals of human solidarity, especially in high-stress situations.

Third, we'll consider the social utility of comic behavior. Why is it so common? Why is it a necessity in high-stress situations and occupations? There are many reasons why we tell jokes: stress reduction, social connection, attacks on persons and institutions, affirmation of freedom, and the need to control unpleasant subjects through words. These reasons will vary with the setting, the prevailing mood, and the people involved, but pervasively there are basic, affirmative human values of freedom, generativity, caring, and pleasure.

The specific purposes of literary comedy regarding medical topics include the following: (1) the naming of difficult subjects, (2) the exploration and change of their meanings and our emotional responses to them, (3) the hypothetical control of such subjects, (4) the exercise of our imaginations, which leads to (5) a sense of agency and freedom, and (6) the creation of supportive comic communities through social rituals using humor.

Fourth, we'll consider applications of humor, practical ways we can care for our health, deal with illness in ourselves or others, improve the delivery of medical care, and maintain, in a preventive sort of way, our health. Despite the saying (and hope) that "Laughter is the best medicine," comedy and humor are not panaceas, and there are many situations where humor is not appropriate. We'll discuss some of the factors governing appropriateness of humor in medical settings.

ITINERARY FOR THIS BOOK

We'll start in Chapter One with my own experience as a cancer patient encountering a clown-like figure in the infusion clinic. We'll discuss some theories and concepts about comedy and tragedy, including scapegoats, the Green World, liminality, domestication, and the differences of healing and curing.

Next we accompany a hospital clown named Vonnie on rounds in two large hospitals (Chapter Two); we'll test some of the theoretical concepts just seen against her work. We identify four qualities of comedy: creating comic community, validating desire, making links to the pleasant past (and future), and enhancing qualities of space.

If Vonnie the clown was gentle, some humor in the ER is not gentle, especially among the caregivers who work there, covering 24 hours a day, seven days a week, especially the dangerous times of Friday night and Saturday night. Indeed ER humor can be quite sarcastic and, in some cases, offensive to outsiders. My example is a running joke about tying up patients (Chapter Three). Although the mood and subject matter are extreme, this joke suggests five aspects of humor: taboo, imagery, esthetic structures (character and story), Freudian attacks, and the themes of aging and death.

These aspects will organize the middle portion of the book (Chapters Five-Nine). For each of these chapters, I'll start with a vignette from a hospital or clinic drawn from real life (with due regard to confidentiality), then discuss jokes from oral and cyber culture that show the pervasiveness of our interest—even fascination—with these five topics.

Chapter Four discusses the wide range of humor, from simple puns to outrageous, ironic humor. I compare the roles of clowns and jokers. I apply the four qualities seen in Vonnie's work to the ER example, and the five aspects seen in the ER to Vonnie. I discuss the usage of sex, issues of appropriateness, concepts of irony and comfort, and the ways comedy can heal us.

Chapter Five focuses on taboo, cultural restrictions on subject matter; humor is one avenue for breaking taboo, thus allowing us to name frightening subjects and, at least for the moment, to deal with them.

Chapter Six discusses images, especially those that show limitations of the human body, with philosopher Henri Bergson as our guide.

Chapter Seven explores character and story, conventional esthetic structures that provide frames for subject matter that may be strange, even bizarre.

Chapter Eight presents humor that attacks persons (often doctors but also nurses) and institutions (hospitals, HMOs, insurance companies) that have power over us. Humor is our weapon for revenge as well as our social criticism, revealing, however indirectly, our deep values for what we believe is fair and health-promoting and what it means to be human, especially when these values are abridged. Freud's book *Jokes and Their Relation to the Unconscious* will provide basic concepts.

Chapter Nine shows how commonly aging and death are on our minds and how we try to deal with our fears about them. In this culture, there is a polarity with youth, sexual attraction, power, and vitality at one pole, and, at the other, old age, sexual decline, weakness, and inertia. This is in some ways an unhealthy and misleading formula, but it is widely used in advertising imagery, and our many jokes on these topics reflect our nervousness and fears about old age.

In Chapter Ten, we explore further examples of hospital humor.

Chapter Eleven returns to the ER for another, more elaborate bit of humor, a running gag in the tradition of office humor about Fluffy, an imagined vicious dog that came into the ER. This bit of comedy encompassed many moods and formats and allowed ER personnel some therapeutic entertainment and catharsis of emotions, until hospital administration shut it down.

Chapter Twelve makes the case for the positive social values when comedy and medicine interact and argues for expanding ways humor can help humanize healthcare and also improve the health of how we live our lives.

While I hope readers enjoy some of the humor in this study, this is not a joke book such as Jeff Rowin's *500 Great Doctor Jokes*.[17] My serious aim is to show that comedy and humor can be an important part of humanizing healthcare in clinical settings and providing a form of preventive medicine in the wider culture. All too often, patients in doctors' offices, clinics, and hospitals are treated in unfriendly and mechanical ways. Comedy and humor can make such places more hospitable and strengthen healing resources in both patients and caregivers. And joking, wherever it occurs, can provide rituals of social solidarity and affirm our imaginative freedom.

Albert Howard Carter III
Social Medicine
School of Medicine
University of North Carolina—Chapel Hill

Chapter One

Comedy, A Cancer Patient, A Clown

W HEN I WAS a visiting scholar at Georgetown University in 1983, I collected my first medical joke, "Doctors Go Duck Hunting" (Chapter Ten) just for fun. Although I had enjoyed hearing and telling jokes, I was primarily an analytic observer in the hospital, with never a thought for a study about comedy and medicine, and certainly never a thought that I myself would be a patient with a serious disease.

When I was diagnosed with cancer in 1995, however, I became an active participant in many things medical. Suddenly I was a sick and worried person entering the strange and complicated world of oncology medicine. Fortunately, I also experienced some of the healing resources of various kinds of comedy.

A CANCER PATIENT'S REPORT:
WHEN IS WHAT HUMOR APPROPRIATE?

In the months before diagnosis, I had a series of infections (eye, throat, skin) that were slow to resolve. Over several weeks my doctor sent me for various tests (allergy, immunology, and more), but these were all negative. This process increasingly frightened me because my health was clearly compromised. Some mysterious form of anarchy threatened my sense of an orderly life. Furthermore, my life history until then was one of robust health. Following the advice of the day, I exercised, ate right, and reduced stress. I was a long-distance runner, participating in 10Ks, a triathlon, and a couple of marathons. That I should be inexplicably sick was not only ironic and anarchic, but totally unfair, even absurd.

I was sent to a cancer clinic, where I felt I was just passing through. I even said to a nurse, "I'm here just to rule out some form of cancer." She smiled, knowing anything was possible. The oncologist took a bone marrow biopsy from my pelvis, and I went home to wait, never dreaming I had cancer.

The phone rang.

"Howard? This is Dr. Peterson. I'm afraid I have bad news. You have a cancer in your bone marrow. The good news is that we have excellent treatments for your disease."

I'm not sure I heard the "good news" or anything else he said. I said, "Thanks, goodbye" and fell on the floor.

When I got my diagnosis of cancer, I was in no mood for jokes. I was distraught, angry, and afraid. I wanted comfort, not amusement, and certainly not outrageous humor. Caregivers at my oncology clinic understood that patients experience psychological trauma in addition to their cellular disease, and they provided various comforts such as snacks and drinks, even valet parking. The space for chemotherapy infusions was a series of pleasant rooms with a large aquarium, TV if we wanted, pretty colors on the walls, and kind nurses wearing scrubs with cheerful colors and designs. Even the waiting room was more like a hotel then anything medical, with up-to-date magazines (what an idea!), books, coffee and tea, as well as comfortable chairs arranged as in a hotel lobby, all cues that we patients deserved a hospitable space and that we were like guests in a luxurious setting, people with leisure and status. Appointments ran on time, a rarity in doctor's offices. Some days I had barely sat down when a nurse called out my name. All these features gave patients the sense of having the comforts of home or a hotel, even though we were in a strange and frightening place.

Especially on my first day of chemo, I was very nervous. Would this hurt? Would I lose my hair? Would I be nauseous? Would I lose mental facility? Would the treatment actually work, or was I headed for disability? Toward death? While my doctor had reassured me on many of these points, some were, of course, unpredictable. Furthermore, I was a complete beginner in this alien world. A common phrase among such patients is, "I felt like I was on the moon," totally estranged from daily, ordinary life.

Most of the time I had no nausea, thanks to anti-nausea medicine, but when I did, it was most unpleasant, making my body feel out of my control. On the other hand, the anti-nausea medicines were themselves sometimes unpleasant. One day I felt as if I'd drunk four martinis very quickly: I was stoned. That day, a friend came to visit and read me a poem he was excited about; the topic (perhaps even the title) was garbage. Ordinarily, I'd be quite interested, but that day I was so intoxicated that I couldn't follow the words, quite an irony for a literature professor.

When irony of life weighs heavily, humor is often unwelcome. "This is no joking matter," we sometimes say about difficult situations. Although a lover of humor for most of my life, suddenly I needed comfort. I needed not a joker but a clown.

A CLOWN IN THE INFUSION ROOM

She came in an unexpected form. Other patients and I were in a large, pleasant room, lying back in our Barcaloungers, receiving our chemotherapy. A small, energetic woman with jet-black hair entered and brought a large tin of cookies around to each of us. Next she offered drinks of various kinds. Then she stood in the middle of the room and announced to everyone, "You know, I lost my hair three times." This was code for I had cancer three different times with three different courses of chemo, each causing my hair to fall out. Nonetheless we could all see clearly that she was healthy and active today. Ten years later I remember her words vividly. Why? Because she gave me a model for survival and vitality beyond the frightening disease and the arduous treatment. She was a person with an exemplary story line of (1) health, (2) sickness, and (3) return to health. Furthermore, in her renewed health she cared about bringing joy and hope to other patients. This woman gave us the image and implied narrative that we could not only survive but also prosper, and she played the role of clown to us, a cheerful and apparently indestructible person. Clowns in the circus fall down and rise again; they strike each other with no damage. Clowns in the rodeo distract a horse or bull away from a fallen rider, surviving danger and helping others do so as well. (For a discussion of rodeo clowns as parallel to physicians, see my book *Our Human Hearts: A Medical and Cultural Journey*, pp. 115-116.)

In Chapter Two, we'll discuss a hospital clown at length, but first I'd like to provide some of the aspects of comedy that will aid our discussion.

COMEDY

One familiar definition of comedy is "a story with a happy ending." This sounds simple, even simplistic, but no less an author than Dante had the same definition for his monumental *Divine Comedy*. In his grand poem, the happy ending came when the central character (also named Dante) joined not only his beloved Beatrice in Paradise but also a whole crowd of saints and Jesus and God too. In the happy ending he found a transcendent unity, well beyond all earthly trials. But before that joy, he had to go through the Inferno and Purgatory. Happy endings are happy, in part, because they come after unhappy passages.

And so it is with comedy in general. We find a basic structure of wholeness, disruption, and regained wholeness, allowing us to experience the emotions of pleasure and joy, perhaps even hilarity. This basic structure and these attendant emotions are the bedrock of all sorts of comedies, those presented on stage, jokes told by the office copy machine, funny movies, and sitcoms on TV. Simple? In one sense, yes, but also primal and therefore powerful, and also the basis for an enormous variety of formulations and uses of comedy, including some very powerful ways that humans communicate with each other, create companionship, and deal with some of the most difficult of human dilemmas, such as trauma, illness, disability, and death.

While moderns typically fear death as a parting, an end, a tragic loss, Christians (and believers of many other faiths) believe in a narrative that goes beyond death to a new unity, a new whole, a new health, which is to say a truly divine comedy. For Christians, it's a New Jerusalem, as described in Revelation or various other visions of heaven. In one sense, death is clearly an ending but also a new beginning for Dante and for many humans, for as long as humans have told stories, made frescoes in ancient tombs, or painted on the walls of Neolithic caves.

Whether secular or supernatural, comedy is a way of exploring some of the deepest meanings of human life, sharing love, and offering hope of another and better life.

COMEDY OF INTEGRATION; TRAGEDY OF SEPARATION

In his *Anatomy of Criticism*, literary critic Northrop Frye suggested that comedy and tragedy focus on the relationship of a character to the society to which he or she wishes to belong.[1] In comedy, the character is accepted or integrated into that society. In tragedy the character is rejected. This concept is immediately clear to any teenager who was not accepted for the team, club, society, or some other deeply desired group. The emotional impact for this teen (and secondarily for the parents) is tragic at the moment of the rejection, even though in a few weeks or even days, the incident may have blown over and life resumed.

FIGURE 1.1: INTEGRATION AND REJECTION

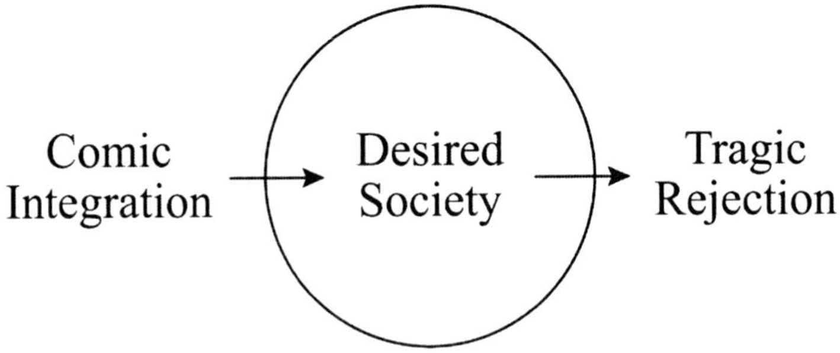

Comic Integration → Desired Society → Tragic Rejection

The teen may find other groups to join in a rebound that we can call comic. Here we see a second movement back to social reintegration, so that it has been often said that "comedy is tragedy narrowly averted." In the full comic trajectory, we move from social balance or stasis "downward" to some kind of disruption or even tragedy, then "upward" to a reintegration and new social balance. We've seen this story a thousand times on TV sitcoms and cop shows, the difference being mainly one of mood; the sitcoms are funny and the cop shows are serious. In recent decades, newscasters have ended their shows, often describing human woe, with "happy talk," their version of reintegration. This "down-then-up" trajectory is the underlying structure of many jokes: we start with a status quo (someone or something walks into a bar), a strange complication ensues, and the punch line provides an unexpected resolution.

For Frye, comedy is a ritual that nourishes us at a deep psychological level. A Shakespearean comedy such as *The Taming of the Shrew* shows us the apparent tragedy of the eldest daughter Kate, who hates men and will not marry, and also her sisters who cannot, therefore, be married, and finally the father, who wants to marry off all three. Petrucchio enters this domestic chaos and slowly wins Kate to marriage

FIGURE 1.2: COMIC REINTEGRATION

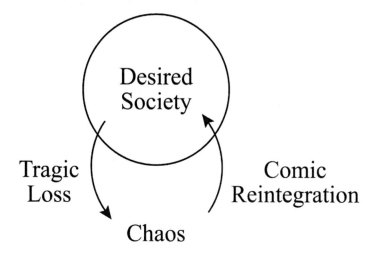

and, by extension, heals her family, even the society at large. Shakespearean comedies imply rituals of fertility because they end in "weddings and beddings" that assure us that the next generations will occur, and society can continue, perhaps forever. Audiences enjoy the dramatic ritual that assures them that male and female can surmount difficulties in order to enjoy sex and procreation and, further, that society will predictably return to a healthy and enduring state.

In summary, we can list attributes of comedy and tragedy in Figure 1.3, remembering that the attributes of tragedy are never far away from comedy, thus providing tension and suspense; indeed a story or play, especially from the Romantics onward, may combine the two.

FIGURE 1.3: FEATURES OF COMEDY AND TRAGEDY

	COMEDY	TRAGEDY
Mythic meaning	Integration	Disintegration
Central social rituals	Wedding	Exile, burial
Sexual meaning	Generativity, birth	Sterility
Symbolic wellness	Health, vitality	Sickness, death
Emotions	Joy, pleasure	Grief, despair
Bodily perception	Pleasure, erotic joy	Pain, suffering
Genres of stories	Comedies	Tragedies

THE NIGHT SEA JOURNEY IN LITERATURE AND IN OUR BODIES

A particular mythic pattern is the *Night Sea Journey*, in which the hero visits some form of the world of the dead but returns alive and healthy to the world of the well. (See Joseph Campbell's discussion in *The Hero with a Thousand Faces*, pp. 90-96, p. 245.[2]) This can be a trip to the underworld, as in classical epics such as the *Epic of Gilgamesh*, the *Aeneid*, or the *Odyssey*. Biblical examples include Jonah and the Whale and even Jesus during his three days in the underworld. In many cases, the journey is linear: down, then up, as we saw in Figure 1.2. In the case of Job, the journey is more existential than spatial: well-being, disaster, well-being again. In such stories the hero starts from a point of normalcy, descends into a world of chaos, and returns to normalcy, often with a "boon of knowledge," in Campbell's phrase. The descent is tragic because of separation, suffering, and various losses. The ascent back to normalcy demonstrates the comic attributes of reintegration, joy, and newfound wisdom and/or appreciation of wholeness.

All who have experienced sickness, injury, heartache, or betrayal know this downward path; to the extent that they have healed from these experiences, they know the upward path as well. If we're seriously sick or injured, our habits, health, and daily activities are all disrupted as well as our sense of order in the world, and even our sense of self. Besides the illness, we have psychological losses such as sadness, loneliness, or anger. Indeed the descent can be psychological only, as in depression or spiritual collapse; traditional terms for these are "melancholia" and "the dark night of the soul." For alcohol and drug addiction, we use the phrase "hitting bottom" before an upward turn toward recovery. Going to sleep each night is a mild, cyclical form of this narrative, ordinarily a gentle version, but sometimes more dramatic if we have nightmares.

The first day of my chemotherapy was the lowest point for me because of the uncertainty, the strangeness, and my fear. As my treatments progressed, I brought more things with me (CD player, all get-well letters and cards, peppermint oil, a sweater, etc.) These were my raft against the Night Sea, a way of domesticating the scary space around my Barcalounger. My wife and friends came to visit me; apparently they didn't mind that I had a needle in my hand and bags of strange liquids dripping into me. Slowly I began to feel part of the community of other patients also receiving treatment. I made friends with the nurses, who began to joke with me. Once my terror subsided, humor was possible.

When we're sick, we feel isolated, apart from the routines of ordinary life. If we're hospitalized, we're physically removed from our homes to a place that may seem very strange, a world apart. Like travelers to a foreign land, patients often discover that they took their healthy life and all its benefits for granted. In this book, I'll call these two worlds "the world of the sick" and "the world of the well." (Susan Sontag speaks of the "kingdom of the sick" and the "kingdom of the well," but these terms seem too regal and hierarchical for me.[3] Who would be the king?) I'll follow Eric J. Cassell, who writes about "the world of the sick."[4] One of the ways of helping sick people feel reconnected to the world of the well is, of course, comedy.

COMIC COMMUNITIES

One very hot afternoon in Orlando, Florida, my wife, my daughter, and I were visiting another family. We had heard that the movie "Raising Arizona" was funny in a quirky way and decided to go see it. The two daughters (young teens at the time) felt it was important to sit as far away as possible from their parents, so they went diagonally across the theater. In between them and the parents were scattered people, mostly of retirement age. During the movie there was not much laughter from the

"Comic Community"

senior citizens in the middle but a lot from the daughters and their parents, two poles separated by the theater's space, but close in comic space as a comic community of six watchers who enjoyed the movie's strange humor and shared in laughter.

While many plays and movies present the comic stories of social integration, audiences themselves participate in another form of social integration. Audiences come together in the space of a theater to watch the show, and they laugh together. They applaud for a play, sometimes even for a movie. People like sharing a pleasurable social experience; subconsciously they feel that their desires and responses to the play are validated because other people are also enjoying the same event. A comic community can be thousands of people at a festival, parade, or rock concert or even millions watching a televised event; it can also be as small as two people swapping jokes in an office hallway or by email.

COMIC COMMUNICATION; THE ROLE OF RITUAL

If the participants have agreed to participate in comedy, that's one thing; if they are strangers (as they often are in medical situations), that's another. In a nursing journal article, Kruse and Prazak write, "Humor can be an effective clinical tool to relieve pain and discomfort and decrease stress and anxiety but only if the intervention is perceived as humorous by the client/patient."[5] They report that there may be differences in perception of humor by age and by gender; other observers points out differences in culture.[6] Sometimes a clown takes a risk, as in the infusion room clown above, and, especially if her humor is gentle, there's a good chance it will work for her audience.

Ritual is one of the ways of matching up the jokers and the audience. The woman in the infusion room was one of many volunteer visitors who brought drinks and snacks; one time we had a barbershop quartet sing to us. Thus patients were used to friendly visitors, even if they were strangers. People who exchange jokes have their own rituals, in person, on the phone, or by email. There are linguistic formulas ("Did you hear about…," "There was this man, see…," "A _____ walked into a bar and…") and clues by gesture, facial expression, and email taglines, all invitations to the Green World of humor, which we'll discuss in a moment.

SCAPEGOATS

By contrast, when a person can be ridiculed by laughter, shunned, exiled, imprisoned, or even executed, the dominating society affirms its own values in rejecting the person who does not measure up. We can consider such a victim a scapegoat, a ritual figure described in Leviticus (Lev. 16.8-10, 20-26). Two goats were taken to the altar, one for sacrifice, the other to take away the sins of the people in its escape. The scapegoat, in being rejected, heals the remaining society. One reading of the crucifixion of Jesus is that he fulfilled both roles, being sacrificed as a paschal lamb to make eternal life possible and also as scapegoat taking away the sins of humanity. In the legal world, we institutionalize, imprison, or even execute people who we judge dangerous to the normal society. In the humor world, scapegoats are figures we reject as inappropriate to our society: we reject them (and the values they symbolize) through derisive laughter. Comedy, in this sense, can be brutal, even tragic, and may include shaming, violence, and/or exile.

A happier variation has the threat of rejection followed by a correction of the deviant individual so that he or she can be reincorporated into society. In the Raising Arizona example, the daughters initially rejected the parents spatially, but later reintegrated them when all six of us together recalled scenes we had enjoyed and we laughed together a second time.

LIMINALITY

Sometimes, however, we're not sure which world we're in, and we float in between. This is a condition of liminality, hovering in a "halfway" existence or standing on a threshold. (Indeed the origin of the word is the Latin *limen* or "threshold.") Perhaps we're awaiting a test result or a diagnosis. A woman wonders whether she's pregnant. The waiting room of a doctor or dentist may seem liminal, a place where an anxious patient wonders, is my health OK? Family and friends wait for answers at an Emergency Room: will the patient be released or admitted to the hospital? A patient in a hospital bed wonders whether he'll get well. A comatose patient in an ICU appears suspended between life and death. All such cases bring doubt and uncertainty; we feel that we've lost our moorings or, if we're family or friends, we worry about the patient and the apparent threat to normalcy, all that we assumed was orderly and certain. In the next chapter we'll follow the hospital clown Vonnie, a liminal figure shuttling between the worlds of the sick and the well and bridging the gap between them.

In some sense, all of us live in a liminal state all of the time, passing from one experience to another, but when health is at stake, liminality contrasts strongly with the order and comfort of our regular routines. Whether we're sick or well, comedy can be a way of suggesting that there are some fixed rituals that can abridge liminality and help us feel at home and in community with other people.

FIGURE 1.4: LIMINAL SPACE

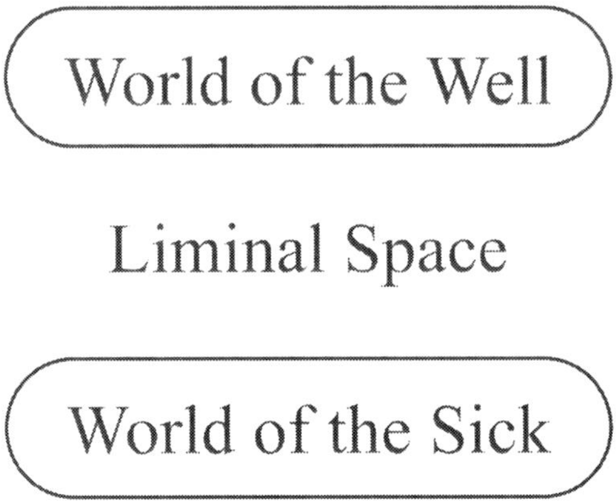

> World of the Well

Liminal Space

> World of the Sick

THE GREEN WORLD AND WORLDS OF OTHER COLORS

Shakespearean criticism uses the concept of the "Green World" to indicate the ideal realms such as the Forest of Arden and other natural or supernatural worlds where lovers can meet (Barber,[7] Frye). In mythic terms, this is a world of freedom and fertility, an Arcadia or an Eden before the Fall. This is a utopia, an ideal place of sunny, blissful pleasure, with no social divisions, no sickness or death, no violence or betrayal, and no ants at the picnic. Sex is innocent and perfect, with the promise of many and wonderful offspring.

Green is, of course, the color of grass and leaves, the renewing colors of spring and the lush verdancy of summer; green is a color that contributes to E. O. Wilson's concept of biophilia, or human love of nature.[8] Before hospitals ruled them out as germy, plants and flowers were a common gift to sick people; now many hospitals have gardens, even labyrinths, as places of reflection and renewal. The Green World is, variously, a world of Pan, Bacchus, and other spirits of nature, an oasis, a place of fertile soil and fertile people, a place of love and procreation, a place of abundant harvest.

All these meanings have important resonances for the world of the well, because the Green World is happy, healthy, and fruitful both for the characters within a comic play or movie and also for audiences watching such comic events. In the comic presentations, the characters yearn for the perfect Green World, but there are also intrusions of the gray world of ordinary life and perhaps even the black world of tragedy, sterility, sickness, and death. In the happy ending of a comedy, all is resolved for the characters, while the audience members have also joined the Green World psychologically, even if their daily circumstances in the normal world are still the same.

People seeing a comic play or telling jokes leave the gray world of ordinary life temporarily to enjoy the Green World of comedy, a touchstone that nourishes them even when they return to domestic chores, bills to pay, and the work world. Two workers telling jokes at a copy machine have made a quick trip to the Green World. Someone working at a computer receives (and perhaps forwards) a piece of humor via email; while this may take less than a minute, it is also a visit to (and an affirmation of) the Green World, and the positive impact can last for hours. The woman who announced that she had lost her hair three times takes me to a Green World every time I think of her.

DOMESTICATION

The root of "domesticate" is the Latin *domus* meaning "house," a place of repose, safety, and pleasure. Idealized, the house is a space for nourishing us, a respite from the trials of the world. As the proverb has it, "A man's house is his castle." In comedy, a home is typically a place for a couple who, despite their conflicts, maintain a symbolically vital and fertile Green World within the domestic and intimate space of their house—the formula for many sitcoms on TV.

French philosopher Gaston Bachelard wrote a book called *The Poetics of Space*, in which he focuses on "images of felicitous space," as opposed to "hostile" space (pp. xxxi, xxxii).[9] For our discussion here, we can think of spatial images of health (houses, dance halls, public squares) as opposed to images of misfortune (junk yards, prisons, cemeteries).

Bachelard shows that our imaginations enjoy images that make sense of our world, in particular, images of the house. He writes "the house is our corner of the world"; it is "our first universe" (p. 4). He continues, "all really inhabited space bears the essence of the notion of home" (p. 5), and "the house shelters day-dreaming, the house protects the dreamer, the house allows one to dream in peace" (p. 6). Finally, there is a maternal aspect of the house: "the house is one large cradle," so that "Life begins well, it begins enclosed, protected, all warm in the bosom of the house" (p. 7).

When we are sick, the qualities and values of our surroundings make a difference: how a hospital room looks, for example, all efficient and institutional. If we leave the hospital and go home, we find it familiar, welcoming, and healing. Perhaps we have a pet, a domesticated creature to comfort us as well. (In my family, a spaniel styled as "Nurse Ben" was loaded onto the beds of persons with colds.)

One of the purposes of comedy is to domesticate the troubling images of illness and injury, to tame them so they can't trouble our minds. We may perceive death as a rabid dog or, through joking, a friendly lapdog.

Healing And Curing

Modern medicine in the West focuses primarily on curing. A broken leg is set and fixed. Pneumonia is cured by pills or IV drugs. A blocked coronary artery is opened or replaced. A cancer is cured by surgery, radiation, and/or chemotherapy. The ideal story line is a complete recovery from the depth of the Night Sea Journey to the level of health enjoyed before the illness or accident. This is the norm, the spoken (or unspoken) performance goal that pervades medicine, especially in society at large. Doctors often don't like partial results ("We regret that a better outcome could not have been achieved"), but we all know that many illnesses (including some cancers and heart diseases) cannot be cured outright and but are, instead, "managed" (in that businesslike term), often for many years. There are also injuries and illnesses that are fatal, for which medicine can provide only palliative care. In this culture, we don't like to talk about death, but we all know that all humans die. Furthermore, we are a society that likes definitive results, such as putting a man on the moon or creating a microchip. When something is fixed, we assume it will stay fixed. This is the realm of curing, an ideal that much of medicine strives for and patients deeply desire.

But there is more to illness than the broken bone, the fever, or the cancerous tumor. (The following comments owe to Eric Cassell's *The Healer's Art*.) Pain registers on sensory nerves, and some drugs can alleviate it. But our intellectual and emotional reactions to our sickness are better described as suffering (or dis-ease), an awareness that we are ill (and incapacitated, annoyed, afraid, and/or angry), often afraid that we might not get better. Wise doctors and nurses know to treat patients' anxiety as well as their specific illness. This is the realm of healing in a wider sense, helping a patient feel whole, even if recovery is slow or full recovery to physical health is not possible. The Hospice movement is an excellent example of helping patients and families heal, even during the dying and death of a patient.

Norman Cousins claimed that watching Marx Brothers movies cured him. Maybe it did. Or maybe his medical treatment cured him. Or maybe the disease ran a natural course and was beaten down by his immune system. Thousands of readers bought his book, fascinated by the prospect that any disease could be cured by laughter; I read it in 1979 and pondered about his success (indeed envied it!) and whether others could emulate him. What an attractive approach: laugh yourself to health;

mind can be victorious over matter; I can think myself well. And, in fact, there are various spontaneous healings, some of them apparently linked to prayer, imagery, mantras, and other psychological events, but these are quite rare, and clearly laughter has not replaced standard medicine in effecting cures. Instead, forms of comedy (including hospital clowns) now complement standard Western medicine, and there are programs for Integrative Medicine at medical schools. Less formally, the well find ways to joke with the sick—as they have for millennia—helping them feel that, although they are sick, they are still human and still part of a comic community that can laugh together in the Green World. More and more we understand that mind and body interact.

MEDICINE

Modern, technological medicine does many wonderful things, some well nigh miraculous. Transplant surgery saves and extends lives. Surgery with robotics, microscopy, and/or laparoscopy achieves marvelous things. Many infectious diseases have been curtailed or even eliminated. America has the best emergency medicine in the world. Care for chronic disease is improving, and many such diseases, as we said earlier, can be "managed," typically with extensive use of pharmaceuticals, which are big, big business. In fact, much medicine is currently driven by institutions with profit motives, such as drug companies, hospital chains, insurance companies, and managed care in general, plus, of course, governmental regulations. Under managed care, doctors typically need to see a minimum number of patients per hour. Taking full histories from patients—let alone friendly conversation—is routinely impossible. The doctor's task is to reach a diagnosis efficiently and, often, to reach for the prescription pad, some of which are printed up in advance with drugs the physician ordinarily uses.

As shaped by TV dramas, the image of medicine has evolved to dramatic interventions in emergency rooms and operating theaters or sudden, brilliant diagnoses. We never see a TV series about routine physical checkups, well baby visits, or physicians advising patients to eat less, exercise more, and reduce stress, all of which are the most cost-effective ways of delivering medical care—preventive medicine as opposed to interventive medicine. Both are necessary, of course, but our social imagery and spending is largely on the interventive side.

Furthermore, we have come to understand medicine as something doctors do to us, because we have lived until something broke down and then needed urgent and expensive care, as opposed to a medical model that encourage us to take more responsibility for maintaining our health, using doctors as consultants. With high-tech

medicine (MD) have fostered this

medical care centralized in big cities and medical schools, we have poor delivery of healthcare in rural areas. With a lack of routine prenatal care, we have, as a nation, poor birth statistics (33rd out of 195 countries, according to UN statistics for 2006). With privatization of health insurance, we have (as of this writing) some 50 million uninsured (before the healthcare reform kicks in) and even insured people often have trouble getting coverage (as shown in the Michael Moore's movie *Sicko*). Medicare and Medicaid have their own difficulties. Dominant economic and political forces still use models from Social Darwinism, assuming that the wealthy clearly deserve their money, while the poor should have known better, should have done better, or should have inherited wealth more adroitly. All these factors are divisive (tragic in our terms), unhealthy for individuals, families, and society at large.

Medicine, we seem to think, primarily treats injury and illness and tries to avoid death; secondarily it sometimes promotes health, happiness, physical and emotional well-being.

NARRATIVE MEDICINE

Narrative medicine is a relatively new subfield that comments on the uses of stories to describe, analyze, and otherwise assess how medicine is conceived and delivered, including bioethical aspects.

Recent books have made important contributions to this growing field, including Kathryn Montgomery Hunter's *Doctors' Stories: The Narrative Structure of Medical Knowledge* (1991) and Rita Charon's *Narrative Medicine: Honoring the Stories of Illness* (2006).[10] Both call for humanizing medicine and offer many useful concept and suggestions for medical care. However, both emphasize interventive medicine and say little about preventive medicine. Both do little with comedy or humor, which, nonetheless, can be a strong resource in humanizing health care of all sorts; their indexes do not include the words "humor," "jokes," or "comedy."

Hunter does refer to residents joking (p. 52) and "grudging laughter" (p. 73), but each time she moves right on to more serious matters. The medical chart has the "cool objectivity of tone" (p. 91), and the stories doctors assemble are not the patients' stories, but "medical plots" with "medical endings" (p. 128). For most of her text, medical knowledge is serious, focused, and instrumental in dealing with illness. In one brief passage she discusses the comic syndrome letter, which satirizes the straightforward syndrome letters in medical journals (pp. 113-117); such comic letters would appeal, of course, to that limited professional community and have no bearing on doctor-patient relations. In a later section, "Healing Narrative" (pp. 131-132), she describes the physician's practice of formulating a medical story that fits the story told by the sick patient; the description is rational, dealing with therapies and possible outcomes, based on a careful interview and physical exam. These are all crucial, of course, and patients and societies should want no less, but we might also want more: healthcare workers who can relate to us as people, through a kind word, a touch on the arm, a small joke—signs of the common humanity shared by patient and healer. Overall, Hunter's approach emphasizes functional utility in the use of serious narrative to create and apply medical knowledge.

In *Narrative Medicine*, Charon also sees the usefulness of stories in the delivery of medical care and the training of doctors. Her focus is on the caregiver in an asymmetrical relationship with a patient who is ill. Her definition of narrative medicine is this: "medicine practiced with these narrative skills of recognizing, absorbing, interpreting, and being moved by the stories of illness" (p. 4). This is all well and good, and the book gives many moving examples of patients she has helped. I'll suggest, however, that a wider perspective would include both the patient-caregiver relationship within a human-to-human relationship, which would be nurtured by small talk, a smile, a joke, a question about the weather, a sports team, or the patient's neighborhood. I imagine Charon uses all of these in her practice, but her book emphasizes healthcare professionals as listeners, "trained confidantes" (p. 78) who enter the worlds of their patients (p. 9), while, it seems, patients do not enter the physicians' world. Furthermore, she writes, patients don't know what is wrong with them: "It is folly to expect that a sick person can tell a professional what the matter is" (p. 99). The caregiver is a "therapeutic instrument," an "agent" with a "duty to witness" (pp.196, 194). These observations emphasize the profound differences between the physician and the sick patient. Charon is more inclusive when speaking of affiliation (pp. 148-151) between physician and patient and between physicians and other healthcare workers, areas where humor and comedy can contribute. Charon makes a compelling argument for narrative bioethics as a wider, more useful, and more insightful frame than principle-based bioethics, and I believe that comedy can play an important role here as well.

In her later book, *How Doctors Think: Clinical Judgment and the Practice of Medicine* (2006),[11] Kathryn Montgomery argues against the notion that physician and patient should operate as friends, because there are times when the physician's authority, objectivity, and efficacy are more important: "Rather than friendship, people who are ill want their physician's committed but disinterested attention as part of ordinary, competent medical care" (p. 183). Instead of being friends, Montgomery argues, they should act as neighbors, in a relationship which requires "the fundamental respect involved in one human being's recognition of another" (p. 185).

The search for the best metaphor for the doctor-patient relationship will probably continue, and probably none will ever be totally adequate, because they include too much or too little. These are terms borrowed from other human relationships and therefore inherently inaccurate, and, furthermore, there is such a variety in the delivery of medical care from routine check-ups to the ICU, from preventive medicine to experimental medicine, from emergency care to epidemiology. My claim is that interactions between doctor (or nurse or tech or unit clerk or med. student) and patient (or family or friends) can often be improved by the use of carefully chosen humor. Indeed Montgomery gives an example of this in some witty banter between a third-year med student and a post-operative patient (pp. 200-201).

There is still more work to be done on the narrative qualities of comedic humor as healing resources; I hope this study helps fill that gap.

So, Who Are We Talking About?

Comedy comes in many forms, as, of course, do people. In the rest of the book, we'll see many kinds of humor used in different ways by different people. Ordinary, healthy people use humor in several ways, for entertainment, for social interchange, for domesticating difficult subjects, and for criticizing things they don't like or find absurd. Humor can range from light whimsicality to savage sarcasm. If we get sick, however, we tend to use a gentler humor for the same purposes. Medical personnel use humor to put patients at ease; it is part of the traditional notion of "bedside manner." When there is a difference in power between caregiver and patient, the humor tends to be gentle. When medical people use humor among themselves, it can be for many of the purposes just mentioned for healthy people, but sometimes there is a dramatic, even raucous humor that deals with tension, stress, and the difficulty of trying to save patients from disease and death. The upshot, then, is that we are talking about everyone, given that we are all vulnerable and mortal.

"bedside MANNer"

Chapter Two

Vonnie, The Hospital Clown

A S A HOSPITAL volunteer, I got to know another volunteer, Vonnie Torbert, a hospital clown. In her curly and bright red wig, she's hard to miss, even from a distance; up close you can read a sign on her vest that reads SMILE PATROL. She visits patients at University of North Carolina Hospitals (UNCH) in Chapel Hill and also at Duke University Medical Center (DUMC) in nearby Durham. When I asked her if I could shadow her on her rounds, she agreed and even rearranged her schedule to accommodate mine.

"Hop Tower"

IVORY - Rapunzel

CLOWNING IN CHAPEL HILL

It is a thoroughly rainy, foggy, and chilly Tuesday, the kind of day that sometimes puts me in a funk. Today, however, I'm happy because I'm going to see a clown at work. I take the elevator up to the seventh floor of Memorial Hospital, called the "bed tower" in hospital parlance. The symbolic aspect of towers interests me. They provide a compact, vertical structure, efficient for architects and caregivers. If the patients' rooms have windows, there are pleasant views over the surroundings, but there are also the visual clues that the patient is removed from the plane of ordinary life, with mythic resonances to Rapunzel imprisoned in her tower.

I'm sitting in the Nurses' Station A in the Rehabilitation Unit at UNCH, where Vonnie and I have agreed to meet. Several nurses greet me and wonder whether I'm doing chair massage today. (At the time, I provided chair massage for nurses once a week). "Nope," I say, "I'm going to follow Vonnie around."

Before long, a large wooden cart with a semi-circular top labeled LAUGH MO-BILE comes rolling across the lobby. Because Vonnie is behind it, pushing it forward, at first I see only her bright red wig with a large puffy blue bow. Then her whole outfit is visible: white pants, boots with stripes of many colors, a blue shirt. Her elaborate rainbow vest sports dangling strings, smiling faces, little animals, doodads of many

sorts, her UNC Volunteer ID, and, front and back, yellow signs reading SMILE PA-
TROL. We greet each other, but she's already spotted a patient being pushed in a
wheelchair on his way back from morning therapy. He looks tired.

"Oh, hi there," she calls out, "and don't you have the most wonderful smile! I'm
going to give you a smile award. Let me put it on you." She rummages in her basket,
from which a rubber chicken is hanging, and pulls out a sticker of a red heart that
reads "You 'R' Special!" She applies it to the man's gown at his shoulder. He's grinning, and trying to take in all this sudden expression of energy and good will. "Now
if you feel a little warmth on the back of this," she continues, "it's because you're
receiving a love transfusion; there's love going into you, from head to toe. It won't
interfere with any of your treatments, and it will keep on working, even if you take
off your lovely pajamas." She gestures to the routine hospital gown the man is wearing. "You have a wonderful day!" she finishes.

And there's another patient being wheeled toward the elevators. She has had
an amputation of the lower leg, a common complication of diabetes. "Oh, are you
sneaking out? I won't tell a soul!" she promises.

"And how about this gentleman," she says, as a man approaches us slowly,
guided by another man, a nurse. The patient walks oddly, because of a left side,
partial paralysis, likely the result of a stroke. Some saliva escapes his mouth and the
nurse dries it with a towel. Vonnie greets the man and gives him a smile award also.
It appears that all of the nurses in this unit are glad to cooperate with Vonnie; they're
familiar with her routines because she's been coming once a week for five years.

We stop at the unit clerk's desk to pick up a census, the daily listing of all patients
and their rooms. The census tells how long a patient has been on this floor, sometimes
as long as the biblical forty days. While Vonnie reviews the sheet, I study her face. As
opposed to some clown makeup with large areas of clown white and elaborate mouth
and eyes, Vonnie's is simple: a heart of red lipstick on each cheek, the same red lipstick on her mouth, red pencil through her eyebrows, and a small heart taped to the
cross-piece of her glasses right between her eyes. With the red wig and red fingernails,
the makeup suggests energy and warmth.

I think it's important for this work that her face shows through: it is not hidden behind a mask of makeup as with some clowns. There are, in fact, people who
are afraid of clowns, as some children are afraid of large, loud Santa Clauses. In an
extreme form aversion to clowns is a pathology called "coulrophobia," or fear of
clowns. In the movie "The Greatest Show on Earth," Jimmy Stewart plays a clown
named Buttons; Buttons is always in makeup because he is, in fact, a murderer. In
Italy, masks were outlawed during the Lenten carnivals because it was a time when

some people in disguise could settle vendettas with knives. There are even jokes today about surgeons in masks committing highway robbery through their fees.

Vonnie is aware that her costume announces her role, for better or for worse. She says, "Sometimes people in elevators won't look at me, and sometimes young people make a snap judgment that I'll be some kind of cliché clown with balloons and stupid jokes. I have to come across more interesting than that!" Signs of her own personhood and humanity show through her limited makeup and also in her voice. When Vonnie talks to patients, she uses a high-pitched, squeaky clown voice, well above her normal speaking register, but when she laughs, her pitch goes down to her normal voice, again revealing a normal, regular person who joins with the patient in the humor of the moment.

Before we get to the rooms, Vonnie speaks with nurse Becky, showing her a card she's made for a patient. There's a photo of a lion (which Vonnie took in Africa) and the notation, "You have the courage of a lion." The patient has been discharged, so Vonnie wants to mail it to him. She offers to pay the postage, but Becky will hear none of that. They mock argue about this trifling amount of money, and Vonnie tells me this nurse is the best nurse in this unit. Becky laughs and carries the lion card away.

Vonnie places the census on the top of the LAUGH MOBILE and studies it once again. She's planning which way to go around the unit and noticing which patients she's seen before and which have been admitted since last week. I look at her Laugh Mobile, essentially a large cabinet on wheels. The top is covered with various baskets and other containers of wands, toys, candy, and rolls of the smile award stickers. The lower part has two large glass doors, through which I can see videos, DVDs, books, and games. Vonnie rolls the cart to the first patient room, sanitizes her hands from a foam bottle mounted there, and whispers to me, "Bed Number 1 has been here eight days." She picks up her basket with the dangling rubber chicken, knocks on the door frame, and we enter.

"Well, say, I see you had your hair done," she says to the woman in the first bed. "Did you fly to Hollywood? That's where I have mine done." (She's using her high, squeaky voice.) "And this," gesturing to me, "is my bodyguard. After all, a good-looking redhead like me can't be too careful. He's a former bouncer at Kmart." And to the woman in the other bed who is wearing a standard hospital gown, she halloos, "Is your nightgown…from Paris? It's so lovely!" The women laugh with Vonnie and begin to talk, explaining why they are in Rehab and what their current treatments are. "I'm so glad you're doing so well," Vonnie says with emphasis. She offers them her stickers and candy. "Now what would you like? Chocolate, Tootsie Rolls, hard candy, gum? I even have non-sugar candy, in case you're diabetic." As we leave, one patient says, "You've made my day," a phrase I will hear from patients several more times over this visit and our next visit at Duke.

As we roll down the hall, we meet people coming to visit other patients. Often they stop and ask if we'll stop in to see a particular person. "Of course," says Vonnie, pulling out the census, "what room?" She'd be going there anyway, but the friends and relatives are happy to have made a request that will be answered—especially in a hospital setting where healthcare personnel make most decisions. The role of friends and family is liminal: they are on a threshold between two worlds, the healthy world where they live versus the world of the sick where their family member or friend must stay—at least for a while. The hospitalized person, now thoroughly in the world of the sick, yearns for any linkage to the Green World of the well. Vonnie's role is to help the two worlds overlap.

When we visit a patient with relatives present, Vonnie asks the patient, "Are these people part of your fan club? Who's the president? The vice president?" She presents such people with a sticker that says Honorary Angel Award. Later she tells me that she can't tell for sure who's married, who is a boyfriend, and so on, but the phrase "fan club" seems to cover all possibilities. It's an ingenious redefinition that expands the concept of the nuclear family to a small comic community. Thus the strange world of the hospital becomes more familial, and the visitors feel a validation from another visitor, albeit one in a wild red wig.

In another room, Vonnie declares that a young man flat on his back (a horse kicked him) needs a "humor tune-up." She takes a wand with a bird head on top and flicks it up and down over his body; the bird head makes a weird squawking sound with each flick. (A label on it reads "Talking Parrot.") "Your humor is in great shape," she informs the bemused patient, "and your smile is just terrific." She presents him with a sticker as part of her spiel. (Indeed, Vonnie herself uses the word "spiel" to describe some of her routines, the German word for "game," suggesting that there are known structures for sharing pleasure.) This particular sticker reads "URAQT," impenetrable as an English word. The young man looks puzzled, but she asks him spell it out letter by letter. He slowly says, "You...are... a...cu...tie" and breaks into laughter.

Another young woman, a car accident victim, can barely move. She complains that she can't reach her legs to scratch them. Vonnie sanitizes a wand and gives is to her so she can reach her legs, saying "I hereby bequeath to you my very special LAUGH MOBILE scratcher!"

In another room Vonnie exclaims, "Oh, I see you're having your gourmet meal.

Was this flown in from the Four Seasons?" The patient, eating uninspired fare, is delighted.

In another room, the woman announces, "This was the first day I walked again. It was just four steps, but I'm just plumb wore out." Vonnie congratulates her and gives her a smile award. She also says, "I know it's discouraging when it all takes so very long. I've had various body parts go down, and I know it seems like forever to get them going again." The woman nods in agreement. "And I'm thrilled," Vonnie adds, offering candy, "to know that you were walking today." Patients often refuse candy on the first offer, but Vonnie always tries again, and frequently they accept it the second time around.

For another visit, Vonnie knocks a loud shave-and-a-haircut rhythm on the door and proclaims, "How's my favorite guy?" before entering and going into her spiel. His head is shaved because of brain surgery; a dramatic red scar curves over the crown of his head. He smiles slowly when she enters. Vonnie is undaunted by his appearance and delayed reactions; she goes right ahead into her routine.

In the hall, one of the visitors to a patient we just saw stops us. "Say," she says, "You don't know how much that meant to him...and to me. It just makes so much difference on a slow, boring day."

"Oh, that's great. I'm so glad," Vonnie says.

When she and I are alone again, she says, "I just love the response. I can't buy what I get here. Basically, I'm a mushy person," and her voice cracks. She wipes her eyes, careful not to smear the hearts on her cheeks. "It's hard to cry with makeup," she says, and suddenly she's laughing.

In the next room, she's explaining about the different colors of foil-wrapped candy kisses she offers: red, green, and silver. "The red ones have twice as much love, the green have spinach, and the silver are regular, but I don't know if they'll keep you regular." Everyone laughs, and the patient chooses red kisses. In the hall, Vonnie tells me that these are Christmas candies some ten months old; a grocery store manager sold her a large amount for a deeply discounted price when she told him how she would use them.

The next time she introduces me as a Kmart bodyguard, she adds, "He was fired because he kept setting all the alarm clocks to go off five minutes apart."

Often Vonnie tells a patient, "Thank you for your smile," a phrase that seems especially effective, because patients often feel passive and useless. When Vonnie affirms that they can still give her something, they feel better about themselves.

After our rounds, we sit in the multipurpose room and I ask her about her clowning. "I was born a silly person," she affirms. "I've found the spot I'm supposed to be in." I ask about her name, "Vonnie." "It's from Yvonne," she says. I think of Yvonne de Carlo, born Peggy Middleton, who came to the screen as the "exotic" movie actress of times gone by. Clearly Vonnie is exotic up here on the seventh floor; there's no one else like her; she's a figure from "elsewhere," or the Green World of clowns and circuses, so that everyone—whether patient, family members, or hospital staff—can recognize her as a familiar, if unusual, figure.

Vonnie has been a hospital clown for over five years; she'd been thinking about the idea when her husband found a news article about a local hospital clown. "I'd love to do that," she said. Vonnie took a two-day course, learning that it was important to make fun of herself and that she innately had the right instincts for clowning. She also learned that her own particular persona as a clown would develop—which she doubted at the time—but later found to be true. For one of her visits, it takes her about ninety minutes to prepare her clothes, makeup, her stocks of candy and other giveaways. Including her travel and a three-hour shift, her total time is about six hours. "I'm real tired when I get home," she says, "but it's worth it."

She continues, "I realize that I make a difference to these patients and families. I'm not a doctor, of course, but I provide the best medicine that I can."

How often have I heard the phrase "Laughter is the best medicine"? We've all heard it, and many believe that there is some or even much truth to it.

Some Cyber Jokes

That evening I check my email and find I have some jokes from a friend:

Health nuts are going to feel stupid someday, lying in hospitals dying of nothing.

Whenever I feel blue, I start breathing again.

In the 60's, people took acid to make the world weird. Now the world is weird and people take Prozac to make it normal.

I read them and laugh. Then I start to wonder, whatever relation do these jokes have to Vonnie's brand of humor? The jokes seem abstract, disconnected from the flesh-and-blood patients I saw today, but my laughter suggests that they work as literary structures, hypotheses using language that engage my imagination. What are the connections between humor in a hospital and humor on the Internet?

Clowning In Durham

Another day we're scheduled for the neighboring city of Durham, historically a tobacco town, but now styled as "The City of Medicine," largely because of Duke

University. I've offered to drive, but Vonnie prefers an itinerary that brings her by my house. When she picks me up, she's already in her costume, and the back seat is full of her gear: baskets, candy, and a wheeled luggage caddy. When we stop at red lights, people stare and she waves back at them. We're headed for her evening shift at Duke University Medical Center—a large, sprawling campus of hospitals, clinics, and research facilities known for cutting edge research. Indeed many very sick people come here from North Carolina, from across the country, and even from around the globe. Vonnie's outfit is similar today, except under her vest she now wears a blue shirt speckled with large orange spiders. We park in an enormous parking structure then make our way to the hospital. Having volunteered here before, I know the nine-story tower to our right is our destination. We're going to visit the cancer service today; I think of Solzhenitsyn's grim novel *Cancer Ward*, from which the protagonist (a projection of the author) finally emerges, a healed man.[1]

We take the elevator to the top floor. I look out a window and see the heliport, complete with red lights and windsocks. Not only are we high above the city of Durham, but we are removed from all the planes of urban life, even the rest of the enormous hospital. Hospital patients are like exiles in any case, and patients looking out the windows know that they are in the highest building around, far above ordinary human life.

There are several levels of care for cancer patients on the ninth floor, and some of the patients are returnees, people who come to Duke regularly for checkups and chemotherapy. Others have recurrences of cancer and are back once more for a stay. Such return visits are often hard psychologically, because Americans believe that when something is fixed, it is fixed, and when you're well again, you're well forever. And of course, returning patients already know the tedium, the boredom, the pain, the routine, the doubts, the expense (money, time, travel), the loss of energy, and even the appearance of other patients who are not getting better. Having regained the world of the well, returning patients may consider returning to the world of the sick a large setback or even a strong clue that death is possible or even imminent.

Perhaps the most dramatic level of care is the Bone Marrow Transplant Unit on the ninth floor. It is not up here just for the view, but because patients receiving marrow transplants have had their own marrow destroyed by chemotherapy and/or radiation to kill their cancer. Because the marrow creates the white blood cells that combat viruses and bacteria, such patients have, basically, no immune systems. Ordinary germs that healthy people routinely deal with might kill a cancer patient here. So the more isolated a BMT unit is, the better it is for infection control. (Similarly, burn units are usually well off the beaten path.) Patients receiving a bone marrow transplant spend a month in a small single room. Typically they are bald from the treatment to kill their marrow. Many have lost weight. More than one person has told me that they look like concentration camp survivors. This is not entirely true, of course, since the starved Jews and others looked far worse, but in today's America of ample food and a variety of hairstyles, the bone marrow patients do look different enough to recall images of World War II concentration camps. After their hospital stays, these patients must stay near Duke another 50 days or so, for a total of eighty-five days away from home.

I hear a loud whirring noise and look out the window. The helicopter is arriving and settling down slowly on the roof. Modern medical helicopters are missionaries of a sort, an extension of the hospital across the skies, covering a large circle with a radius of some 250 miles. These machines are marvels of design and efficiency; flight nurses (often small of stature) care for one or two patients in a narrow space. Medical helicopters were an offspring of the Korean war, landing where no fixed-wing aircraft could, and quickly taking the wounded to a mobile army surgical hospital, or—as we all know from the movie or TV series—a MASH unit. From this the term "mede-vac" entered common language. Along with helicopters for news stations, medical helicopters are familiar and comforting sights, a decentralization of hospitals that make us feel, subconsciously, more safe and secure, since they can land on streets, highways, parking lots, fields or Interstates and whisk the injured away to a trauma center. I see medical helicopters now and then from my house. If the helicopter is going east or west, it's Duke's; if it's going north or south, it's UNC's. They suggest that a person needs help and that help is on the way.

Vonnie and I stop at the office for Oncology Recreation Therapy, where I meet Kristy Everette, CTRS (Certified Therapist Recreation Specialist), who helped arrange my visit. She's talking with another volunteer who will soon be taking out a hospitality cart with coffee and snacks. Kristy's office is crowded with handbooks, games, videos, music cassettes, and other resources to brighten a patient's hospital stay. Vonnie and Kristy go over the census, which Kristy has carefully annotated for each patient. She knows where they're from, what relatives are visiting, and where they stand with medical procedures. Vonnie knows a lot of this, having seen many of them in previous weeks. As she pushes the Duke LAUGH MOBILE out the door, she pauses to make an addition to her curly red wig, a spray of wires that appears to shoot out of her head like the spray of feathers on the head of the Muppet Big Bird. On the end of the wires are metallic disks like coins; these flash and twinkle as they catch light from the fluorescent lights overhead.

We push through double doors to enter a short hallway; air rushes against us because the pressure differential is designed to keep germs out. The wall displays photos of patients who have "graduated" from the Bone Marrow Transplant Unit. Vonnie and I sterilize our hands from foam containers on the wall and push through the next pair of doors. As we enter the unit, a nurse greets Vonnie; clearly they know each other. The nurse doesn't know me, however, and looks at my temporary ID badge and asks me why I, a complete stranger, am visiting. I explain.

Vonnie parks the LAUGH MOBILE outside one of several doors that line the hall. I think of sleeper rooms on a railroad car. "Can you sing?" Vonnie suddenly asks me. Is this woman psychic? (I'm a trained singer, accustomed to being on stage with choirs and choruses, but I've never had a venue like this.) I say that I do.

She explains, "Well, it's this patient's birthday, not the regular one, but because she got transplanted today they call it 'day zero.' For the patient, it's like a birthday of a second life after cancer. So how about singing 'Happy Birthday' for this patient?" I agree.

She knocks at the door, and someone says, "Come in."

The room is small but pleasant, with a window to the outside. A young woman, entirely bald, is in bed, her mother and a young man smile at us, recognizing Vonnie from earlier visits. The young man, clearly the donor, has bandages on each forearm, because his blood was drawn from him, sent through a machine—which removed the cells needed for the transplant—and returned to him. Then the cells were injected into the patient. Vonnie introduces me as a baritone from the Metropolitan Opera, flown in this afternoon for this special birthday. I start to sing the standard "Happy Birthday" song, progressively adding vocal flourishes and lavish gestures. During my opening notes, I wonder whether I might be bothering a patient next door but decide—what the hell—that's exactly why we're here today, to bring messages from the outside world to this remote setting. My immediate audience grins during my song and applauds at the end.

Vonnie asks about the transplant, and all three explain how it went, picking up from each other in a round-robin chorus. With any serious illness, a whole family is commonly involved and, in this case, a brother gave cells to his sister. Vonnie gets out her Honorary Angel Award sticker for the brother, and the mother grabs her purse to show that she already has this sticker and has put it on her purse. Nonetheless she gladly accepts another award.

In another small room a young, bald man is working on a laptop computer with some paper strewn over the bed. From a few feet away, I can see that the pages are alike, printouts of some sort. Vonnie asks him about his treatment. "It's my second transplant," he says. "I sure hope this one works." I'm moved by the faith and confidence of these patients. Vonnie asks about the pages. "Oh, I'm still working; I need to review and summarize these data for my company." For this patient, work is possible through cyber links to the outside world; I imagine this helps him feel that he is still valuable and capable, still linked to the world of the well.

We leave the BMT unit through the pressurized hallway with two sets of doors and head toward the "floor," a ward for a variety of cancer patients with a variety of treatments. As with many specialized acute-care services, the BMT unit is a highly focused place, suggesting a dramatic urgency to help very sick patients. The "floor," by contrast, seems more relaxed.

But first we sit down for a few minutes and do some quality control on Vonnie's store of chocolate, consuming several pieces. This is the only time we'll sit over the three and one half hours of our visit this evening. Some visitors pass by in the hallway. "How about some candy?" Vonnie pipes up and heads toward them with her basket. "Who are you visiting? What room? We'll stop by for sure." It's now dark outside, but hospital hallways are lit night and day.

As she pushes the LAUGH MOBILE into the oncology unit, Vonnie tells me, "Some patients are hours or even days away from home, so visitors for them are rare, even nonexistent. I've had people crying up here, because not a soul has come to see them."

Unlike the BMT rooms, these are regular hospital rooms, larger and with more freedom of access for visitors and nurses. The hallway is busy with nurses, doctors, and visitors, even patients getting some exercise, some walking with IV poles, some walking with a large wheeled support. A sign on the wall tells how many feet make up a trip around the triangular hallway, and what fraction of a mile this equals. Typically, patients who walk more heal faster.

Our visits proceed much as they did in the Rehab Unit at UNC. Vonnie knocks and, if invited, enters and goes into one of her spiels. She has her candy, her stickers, and her quick wit to deal with whatever she sees. If she notices a Bible or a cross, she'll say, "I'll keep you in my prayers." Patients have a wide range of religious inclinations, of course, so she mentions prayer only if there's a solid clue.

At another room, there's a routine I haven't heard before. Vonnie holds out her plastic stethoscope and proclaims, "Hi there! I'm Dr. Silly. I'll be replacing your doctor tonight; he fell down and got a bloody nose. What can I do for you besides making you completely well? Chocolate? Life savers?" The patient is puzzled at first but quickly perceives the comic spirit and begins to laugh.

Amidst all of our cheery visits, I see signs of serious and exacting work. A large chart on a wall lists dozens of drugs horizontally and vertically, marking incompatibilities where they intersect. Another posted notice lists levels of duties for the various ranks of the CNAs (Certified Nursing Assistants). Another memo gives guidance to what may be written in order to avoid errors in administering drugs: there are to be no "trailing zeros" (never 2.0 but always 2) and no "naked decimals" (never .4, but always 0.4). Vonnie's work also depends on attention to details and protocols (confidentiality, germ control, who can eat sugar), although she has more latitude in how to meet patients' needs creatively. In one room, no visitors are allowed so she stuffs candy into a latex glove and pitches it across the room to the patient's bed. In another room, the bed is empty. Where is the patient? We don't know, but Vonnie leaves a teddy bear with a note, "Sorry I missed you. —A Beautiful Redhead." Her mood is so consistently upbeat, no matter what the visual clues of her patients' illnesses may be—from bald heads to sallow skin color, from bandages to medical equipment, from missing limbs to bright red scars.

There's one room that we skip entirely, a lead-lined room. It has a huge metal door reminiscent of a prison. This grim chamber is for a patient who has been given a particular radioactive drug to destroy cancer cells; he or she must stay in the room until no longer hot and a danger to others. This isolation or quarantine seems an extreme version of the separation of a sick and toxic person from the ordinary world of the well. Since there's no patient's name posted by the door, I feel some relief that at least for today, no one is sequestered there.

When we finish all the rooms, it is thoroughly dark outside. We return to the recreation therapist's office, where Vonnie annotates the census she's been using and leaves a note for Kristy. Vonnie puts the LAUGH MOBILE away, packs up her stuff, and we make our way back to the parking deck. It's been a long, intense evening, and we're both tired. As she drives me back to my home, we don't say much, but I think we've both seen and enjoyed the power of her work with patients.

BRINGING THE CIRCUS INTO THE SICK ROOM: INTERPRETING VONNIE

Vonnie is immediately recognized as a cheerful clown, a familiar social role. (We're speaking here of the tradition of the Harlequin or happy clown, not the Pierrot Lunaire or sad clown.) Whether Vonnie is in an elevator, a neighboring car, a hallway, or a hospital room, everyone knows her by the wig, clothes, and makeup; she's immediately seen as someone who entertains, makes jokes, and brings a vital energy. People associate her with a circus, seeing a clown on TV, or enjoying one at a child's birthday party. What are the implied values of experiencing Vonnie? I suggest the following four.

1. Creating a Comic Community

When Vonnie enters a room, she brings her mini-circus with her through her appearance, her clownish voice, all her props, and, of course, her wit in spirited conversation. She includes everyone present, the patient, friends and family, any nurses, even me. A patient who may have felt lonely, isolated, or sad (in short, exiled from ordinary life) is suddenly in a whirlwind of energy, attention, and caring, part of an ad hoc comic community. All present are, to use Max Eastman's phrase, "in fun," sharing the mood and the play, wit, and freedom of the moment; they forget the medical milieu with all the implied threats and separations, and they enter the Green World of comedy.

2. Validating Desire

Vonnie allows people to feel positive desires and express them. She congratulates patients on their smiles or their medical improvement. A veritable cornucopia, she rewards them with several kinds of candy. She leaves a teddy bear for one patient and gives a wand for scratching to a young woman. Vonnie validates anything patients say, responding to the meanings and emotions of their words. If they express concern, doubt, or worry, Vonnie affirms them without question or hesitation. In the hospital world, patients' personal needs are often deemed less important than their medical needs and the needs of healthcare personnel. When Vonnie visits, however, the patient has freedom to speak and be heard, a focus for Vonnie's loving attention. For a patient seeing Vonnie a second or third time, the values are even stronger: *I know Vonnie, and she knows me; we always have a good time together.* Furthermore, Vonnie has the ability to voice unspoken desires of patients, basic points that they are too shy or too polite to mention, such as the monotony of hospital food.

While much of her humor is gentle and friendly, there are a few bits of attacking humor, for example, the fun made of hospital gowns and food. When she comments on women's hair, Vonnie indirectly refers to the difficulty in staying groomed and attractive. Her mention of a doctor falling down and receiving a bloody nose may represent a patient's unspoken anger at being captive in a hospital and rarely seeing the doctor who, it is hoped, can deliver wellness. And there was a brief reference to "regularity," suggesting challenges in bowel function when a patient is bedridden for days or even weeks.

3. Links to the Pleasant Past (and Future)

Rolling her LAUGH MOBILE along, Vonnie brings her own circus with her, and circuses are, for the vast majority, known and pleasurable events in patients' life histories.

Vonnie, therefore, gives a link to happy times in the past, recontexting a patient away from the current gray world of the hospital to the timeless Green World.

The circus is a place full of spectacle: athletes wearing scanty, form-fitting costumes, color, lights, music, exotic animals, popcorn, cotton candy, and magnificent spatial organization of three rings horizontally plus multiple levels of height (trapezes, high wires, etc.), all under the apparent control of the ringmaster. We are dazzled by the risks athletes take and thrilled when they are safe. Similarly, we see clowns fall down and rise up for further antics. If a clown can surmount threats of all sorts, so can a hospital patient.

For many patients, this notion may be subconscious, but I'm suggesting that clown Vonnie represents a version of the Night Sea Journey; she is an exemplar that allows them to imagine that the descent of their illness will be followed by the rise of their recovery. Even if death is an outcome, for persons of religious faith the "recovery" is a second life beyond this one. Some years back I wrote an article that suggested the Living Will was a conceptual variation on the Night Sea Journey, a kind of warm-up for death.[2] Although it's a hypothetical trip on paper, my wife and I found it disturbing as we considered whether we'd like ventilators, full codes, renal dialysis, and the like if either of us were very, very sick. Even with the work of Hospice, Elisabeth Kübler-Ross,[3] and a raft of thanatology studies, there are still many taboos about death in this culture. In my hearing, Vonnie never mentioned death, but in her performance she embodied the opposite: possibilities of return to the world of the well beyond the hospital. Her repeated visits symbolized that she could enter the hospital many, many times, and leave each time—thus a model for patients lying in bed. At one point, she mentioned to a patient that she had had "various body parts go down" and was now clearly back in business, a person who triumphed over illness. Through all this, the patient is allowed to imagine a future beyond the hospital, so that the hospital stay is now symbolically enclosed between two healthy times, ideally a blip on a larger, happier trajectory.

4. ENHANCING QUALITIES OF SPACE

We've considered reorientation in time, reconnecting patients with a pleasant past and a probable future; we may also consider reorientation in space. Following Gaston Bachelard, we can understand space as having qualities, meanings, associations, or moods. We know the difference between a stay in a prison and a picnic on a river bank. We know the difference between being able to move freely and being enclosed in bandages or a cast, or frozen by a locked-in syndrome, dramatically shown in the recent book and film "The Diving Bell and the Butterfly."[4]

If a hospital room seems utilitarian, impersonal, and sterile, like a lab or even a prison, the patient may feel like a lab rat or a prisoner. In the last few decades, however, hospital designers have given more thought to colors, graphics, murals, curtains, and the like to make the space seem more like a hotel or a spa. Family and friends bring in photos, cards, and balloons in order to make a generic room personal, special, festive, even more like home. Such domestication is another way of building comic community, and nurses and others will ask patients, "Oh, is this a picture of your dog/grandchild/house?" When space is domesticated, the patient feels more like being at home, and the psychic distance from actual home is diminished.

In Vonnie's work, the hospital room is symbolically a venue for a traveling circus, a worthy place to set up the tent, to lead in the elephants, and to play the music. In the patient's mind, the qualities of the room change when Vonnie enters the room. Even after she has moved on, the various keepsakes (stickers, candy, a teddy bear) keep her visit alive in patients' imaginations.

In sum, Vonnie brings energy, jocularity, and kindness in a traditional character of a clown; she comes from the outside world of (relative) order, predictability, and pleasure. Patients can see themselves in a symbolic circus, a place of joy, action, and shared laughter. While this may be temporary—ten minutes, say—her impact lasts longer than that, especially for patients hospitalized long enough for repeat visits from her. These visits are not paid for or earned in any way; they are gifts. In a religious sense, they are acts of grace. Whether patients realize this or not, they understand, at some level of consciousness, that there is a personal validation of them in each visit: they are worth the effort, focus, and personal attention of a hospital clown who comes to their very own rooms—no matter how they look or feel, no matter how difficult their medical condition may be—in such a way that "makes their day."

These four qualities will help us interpret other events from hospitals and clinics and also in the jokes from the oral and cyber worlds that treat parallel subjects. Specifically they may help explain the success of hospital clowns in other clinics and hospitals. A German study reports more positive attitudes among psychiatric patients after one clown visit per week for six weeks, and an Italian study reports that pediatric patients being readied for surgery were less anxious when visited by a clown.[5] Selena Clare McMahan has studied hospital clowning from the inside, volunteering or working internationally with various organizations including Clowns Without Borders. She observes that "the hospital staff is there to treat the part of the patient that is sick; the clowns are the only workers in the hospital there to connect with the part of the patient that is healthy—their spirit and imagination. Even someone on the verge of death can still smile and make a joke."[6] As to the notion of agency, she writes, "one of the very most important benefits of hospital clowning is the control it gives to the patient. A sick child in a hospital is someone with no power—she is small, she is sick, people are doing things to her body, and she cannot leave or tell them to stop. A clown arrives and suddenly there is someone in the hospital who will do what the child asks for."[7] Similarly for an elderly patient: "He is physically trapped in an unfamiliar environment where other people are in control of his body, his schedule, and his future. He is without power and often even more ignored than a child would be. The clown arrives in this environment, addresses his healthy spirit, and gives him control of the interaction."[8]

CLOWNS—HEALTHY, INDESTRUCTIBLE SURVIVORS

The word "clown" relates to the word "clod," the earth, especially seen in the tradition of rodeo clowns who protect cowboys from being trampled in an arena of dirt. Circus clowns are athletes; they fake fights, take falls, and make tumbling moves. Clowns are healthy, apparently indestructible, although their costumes—with goofy polka dots, big ties, big shoes—hide their physical prowess. Their makeup of big eyes and big smiles makes them appear permanently happy. Similarly, Vonnie always appears happy, regardless of how a patient appears, and she'll discuss any topic, even a patient's fears. She's flexible in matching her comments to a patient's; her verbiage is free-form, a kind of improv comedy or even street theater that matches the cues she takes from her patients.

While Patch Adams' work is perhaps the most well known, there are other hospital clown programs. Clown Care, for example, is an outreach program of Big Apple Circus that works with eighteen pediatric facilities across the US. Some ninety specially trained "clown doctors" visit children in both inpatient and outpatient units, including intensive care, emergency room, physical therapy, bone marrow transplant, pediatric AIDS, and hematology/oncology. A recent issue of *The New Yorker* carries a full-page advertisement for the Big Apple Circus Clown Care program (November 23, 2009, p. 121). A color photo shows a clown holding a stethoscope on the top of a child's head. The end of this instrument is actually a plumber's helper, and the child is smiling. Accompanying text says that clowns "tend to the important business of creating a smile, a laugh and lightness in the room. And with that comes a true feeling of healing and hope."

There are also other ways the healthy world can embrace and comfort hospital patients, reminding them that they still have links to the ordinary world of the well: architecture that seems like a hotel or a spa, colorful murals, fountains, gardens, and labyrinths. Nurses' scrubs often sport cheery designs. Such resources are helpful to family and friends as well, giving them a bridge between the two worlds.

MORE CYBER JOKES

The next day I find some more jokes in my email.

Why do people point to their wrist when asking for the time, but don't point to their crotch when they ask where the bathroom is?

Why do OB-GYNs leave the room when you get undressed if they are going to look right up there anyway?

These two jokes have sexual content different from the humor of Vonnie's visits. How are we to understand them? What role do they play in health and healing?

And what about the robust, raucous, even weird humor of the Emergency Room? How can that relate to the gentle, validating humor of Vonnie? In the next chapter, we'll see what we can learn from humor in the ER for occasions when nurses must tie patients to their beds.

Chapter Three

Party Time!

A Ritual of Black Humor in the Emergency Room and One Forty-Year-Old Joke

F OR A DOZEN years or so I was a volunteer in the Emergency Room of a large urban hospital, working out of the Chaplain's office one afternoon a week. My job was to provide pastoral care, such as visiting patients, making phone calls to families, and arranging their visits. Sometimes I did errands and small chores in the ER: changing the sheets on the gurneys between patients, taking specimens to the lab, or going to Medical Records or the Pharmacy. Because I had interests in medicine since my youth—indeed I thought for a while I might be a doctor—the ER was a good assignment for me.

I didn't become a doctor. Although briefly pre-med in college, I changed my major to literature, which seemed to be another good way to learn about people. I was still interested in medicine, however, because the medical encounter was an occasion where some of the deepest aspects of humanity could be observed, both in the suffering and anxiety of patients and in the efforts of healers to offer technical skill and human empathy. When the field of literature and medicine emerged in the early 1980s, I knew I had a natural home for my research and writing. Literature—even the oral tradition of jokes—is one approach to studying patients and caregivers (who are inevitably, at some times, patients themselves).

As practiced in American hospitals, the culture of medicine is well prescribed by professional codes, ethics, standards of care, and, of course, laws. Even as hospital volunteers, we were taught about sterile fields, AIDS, confidentiality, cross-cultural sensitivity, and more. After our six weeks of training, the volunteers requested the areas they'd prefer to work with; because of my E.M.T. background the Emergency Room was my choice. Further, I wanted to be part of the *action*, to see some of the extremes of human experience and the intensity of medical care brought to bear as quickly and accurately as possible—the kind of action that TV shows offer to eager audiences. Indeed my ER received patients via ambulance, rescue unit, helicopter, taxis, and private cars. Even walk-ins. Since we were also a Level II Trauma Center, we saw a wide variety of patients from a catchment area some 250 miles in every direction. What's not shown on TV, however, are periods of boredom, the stocking of supplies, and patients waiting to be seen, waiting for lab results, or waiting for a bed upstairs.

Many strange and upsetting things came through our doors. Even after several years—when I thought I'd seen everything—each month brought a new surprise about ways humans could be sick or injured. We saw people who fell down in their homes or jumped off bridges, also people who lost their memory. There were victims of chainsaw accidents, house fires, car wrecks, or lightning strikes; cases of delirium tremens, suicide attempts, overdoses from street drugs or prescribed medicines; also hallucinations and other psychotic breaks (one woman assured me she was from another planet). Some patients had heart attacks, asthmatic crises, or high fevers. There were victims of muggings, rape, shootings, stabbings, and other crimes. Many of these were treated and released. Many were stabilized and then sent upstairs for further treatment. Sometimes a patient died in our ER. Occasionally we had a precipitous birth, the baby coming so fast that the mother could not be transported upstairs to Labor and Delivery. One day we all heard the plaintive cry of a newborn coming through the curtains. Soon the nurse stuck her head out and announced, "It's a boy," and we all applauded—a small, ad hoc comic community.

In my observation, the nurses, doctors, technicians, unit clerks, and administrators were wonderful in dealing with the sick and wounded who entered their doors. Such hospital personnel were underpaid, overworked, and often unrecognized. I salute their professionalism, courage, and faithfulness. I also enjoyed their humor.

Humor In Extreme Situations

Folklore says a man about to be hung joshed, "This will surely teach me a lesson." Accordingly, we call this sort of humor "gallows humor."[1] More broadly, people make jokes about desperate situations, in part to put language to them, in part to show freedom in the face of overwhelming forces. In modern times, the book, movie, and TV series *M*A*S*H* showed such humor to wide audiences in the US and abroad. Working in very difficult conditions, the Army doctors and nurses treated the wounded but also cracked jokes, made puns, and performed practical jokes, all to keep their own sanity intact. (By the time of the movie and the TV shows in the early 1970s, the humor that attacked military governance and war's absurdity was easily transferrable by viewers to the ongoing Vietnam War.) More recently, Lee and Bob Woodruff wrote, "Gallows humor has its root in the quest for sanity. When the situation is so black, so dark, that grief or fear threatens to overwhelm, there is nothing like a good joke or two to resuscitate hope" (*In an Instant: A Family's Journey of Love and Healing*, p. 64).[2]

It's common knowledge that ER workers have unusual senses of humor, but they are not alone, since other subcultures of medicine—and especially services where stress is pervasive, such as intensive care units, surgical services, and burn units—have their own language of jokes, humor, and comic play. For such caregivers, this humor is not strange or weird; rather it is normal and necessary. (It's also true that they have gentle, "normal" humor, but outsiders are usually interested in the unusual humor.) Such humor is a way of dealing with the pressures the workers face daily, pressures that cause many to transfer to calmer areas of the hospital, to clinics, or even to other professions. Humor is a way of saying, "Let's get this straight: it's our patients who are sick and injured, while we, the caregivers, are well. We need to maintain our wellness so that we can help them." Similarly, other high stress occupations have their own unusual humor: journalism, music, and sports, to name a few.

As my friend Colleen Adomaitis, then working as a phlebotomist, put it, "Any time you're providing critical care, there's lots of pressure. I'd have to wait my turn to draw blood on a patient who coded while the team swirled around him. When my turn came, it could be easy to panic, to freeze up. Everyone knew this, of course, and often someone would make a joke to set me and others at ease so that things would go smoothly."

The Emergency Department of UNC Hospitals has a large waiting room with numerous official plaques explaining, in English and Spanish, patients' rights for treatments. On another wall is a unique, unofficial plaque with the following hand-lettered text:

> If You Are Waiting
> Possibly you may see us laughing
> > or even take note of some jest
> > but know that we're giving your loved one
> > our care at its very best.
> There are times when tension is highest;
> > there are times when our systems are stressed;
> > and we've discovered humor a factor
> > in keeping our sanity blessed.
> So, if you're a patient in waiting
> > or a relative or friend of one seen,

don't hold it against our smiling.
It's a way to handle this team.
Sincerely
The staff
UNC ED
Emergency Nurses Day
1999

Although unsophisticated in its expression, this statement is a credo of sorts: a declaration that caregivers need humor in order to maintain themselves and the health of their entire team, a comic community within the Emergency Department.

To outsiders, ER humor can easily appear demeaning and condescending. One day one of our patients was seizing, thrashing around on his bed. "What's up with M-3?" I asked his nurse, indicating that patient in medical bed number three. "Oh, looks like the backstroke," Ted replied, before explaining the actual medical condition. Was Ted disrespectful of his patients? Perhaps so, to outsiders. But I knew that Ted was an excellent nurse and understood that his comic quip expressed his helplessness and anxiety about a patient he could not immediately cure. Like the doctors and everyone else in the unit, he had to wait until the drugs would take hold and help that patient. Or perhaps he was waiting on lab results.

Some humor is derisive and condescending. While observing with a fire department during my E.M.T training, I heard the phrase "model citizen" applied to street people. I also remember visiting another hospital in a large city and hearing a senior doctor speak deprecatingly of the "knife and gun club." By this sly phrase he meant wounded patients (mostly male, typically intoxicated or on drugs) who came to the Emergency Room on Friday and Saturday nights from the section of town where poor people lived. To me, the phrase suggested a smug refusal on his part to have empathy for such people, and I did not wish to join his comic community. By contrast, the ER humor I observed at my hospital—while sometimes dramatic and absurd—was in the context of providing good care for patients. (Perhaps if I'd have seen the "knife and gun club" doctor at work caring for patients, I'd have a different opinion of his phrase as well.)

Medical humor can be unusual in its harshness or as ordinary as office humor anywhere: the ritual exchange of jokes, the playful postings on bulletin boards and email, the running gags, and the shifting of materials (paper, photocopies, staples, Post-Its, markers) from a common to a comic use. Many topics, such as bosses, lack of resources, and company policies, are routine and predictable. Indeed, I've seen the same joke posted backstage at a major symphony orchestra and in a radiology suite: *The beatings will continue until morale improves.*

PARTY TIME! COMIC LANGUAGE FOR A DIFFICULT ACTION IN THE ER

A desk in the charting station contained a large drawer, the standard size for files. Instead of files, however, there was a tangle of belts, straps, and cuffs padded with wool; these were made of thick tan leather with stainless steel hardware. Occasionally a nurse would pull open the drawer to remove some of this equipment in order to restrain a patient on the order of a physician. Other nurses passing by would utter a ritual comment of Party Time! either as statement or a question. Here are some of the variations of the statement and response:

"So, party time."…"Uh huh, you bet."

"Party time?"…"Not hardly."

"Hey, party time!"…"Oh yeah, for sure. Want to join in?"

The first time I heard such language I was startled. Had I heard her right? The next few times taught me that this was a standard utterance for this working group; it seemed to symbolize some set of social values. What could Party Time! possibly mean?

Party Time! was code for "I see that you're going to tie a patient to the bed, and I know that you and I both hate doing this." The underlying ironic metaphor compares restraining a patient to wildly inappropriate images of sexual play, particularly domination and submission, presumably by adults who have chosen to play such roles or, even worse, for an episode of captivity, torture, and/or rape. The ER reality, of course, is just the opposite: a patient who is violent or deranged enough to be a danger to himself (and it was usually a male) or to others must be restrained for the safety of himself and anyone near him.

One day a patient in a one-point restraint wrenched his hand loose and tried to hit a nurse. All nurses were immediately upon him, and soon he was in four-point restraints (both hands and feet tied). This was a rare event, but such a threat is always possible, especially from drunk, drugged, or mentally ill patients. Party Time! reflects indirectly the nurses' distaste for the necessity to limit a patient's freedom severely by tying him up. When a policeman handcuffs a wounded suspect to the bed, there are sufficient legal reasons, and it is the policeman, not a nurse, who does the deed.

While they have differences in sentence structure and mood, the statements and responses all work the same basic ritual affirmation: *we*—right here making jokes—

are so well that we might be involved in a sex party, but the patient about to be restrained—over there, implied, generic—is sick, tragically sick. We are part of a comic community, different from the patient, an outcast whom we have removed from society.

To be tied up is an extreme instance of spatial limitation and an exercise of power of a person or persons over another. It takes away freedom, choice, and humanity. We tie up prisoners, dogs, and farm animals. In the past, slaves were shackled. More recently, images of tied-up (and otherwise abused) prisoners of Abu Ghraib and Guantanamo have disturbed viewers around the world. Such restraints symbolize, at best, responsible control over a person or animal; at worst, the intent to humiliate and harm.

The medical chart will read something like "pt. placed in two-point restraints at 14:50 per doctor's order." This formulation minimizes the personhood of the patient ("pt.") and also the agency of the nurse, by using the impersonal passive tense. The time is styled on a twenty-four hour clock, which suggests scientific and military resonances of objectivity and control. Further, the medical phrases "two-point restraints" (usually both hands) and "four-point restraints" are euphemisms in technical language that avoid the more direct, obvious, and troubling phrase "tying up hands and feet." "Restraint," as opposed to "leash" or "shackle," seems to be a gentle word. Indeed much of medical terminology—with formal Latin and Greek roots—has associations of power, elitism, and advanced education; such language, of course, has been a satiric target for centuries, as we'll see in Chapter Five.

By contrast, the phrase Party Time! has the promise of erotic joy, freedom, and adventure; we may recall baseball player Nuke LaLoosh, who allows himself to be tied up in Annie Savoy's bed in the movie "Bull Durham." In the ER, by contrast, Party Time! ironically emphasizes the profound losses of sexual freedom, pleasure, and self-expression when a patient is tied to a hospital bed. To tie up a fellow human being is to commit a violent act, even for the sake of avoiding other violence. Such fellow humans, restrained, are mirrors to hospital personnel, who may imagine some version of "There but for the grace of God go I."

For all these reasons, nurses detested having to visit the drawer full of restraints, and Party Time! became a sarcastic acknowledgment of the meanings and emotions implied. It is, in brief, a code to express the underlying disgust, resentment, sadness, even anger at having to perform such an act. We sometimes call macabre humor such as this "black," portraying a dark world that seems, at first glance, far from the Green World of comedy.

I should add that I have no idea how many nurses participated in the ritual, given that three shifts kept the ER open 24/7/365. Perhaps this particular comic community was only six or ten people who knew each other well. (Or more?) For our purposes, however, the actual number doesn't matter, since the ritual apparently had meaning for the nurses I observed. Nor did I ask any of the nurses what they felt about the phrase. I would guess that they didn't give it any in-depth interpretation, and they just performed the ritual without speculation as a part of their working society.

Aspects Of Jokes, Humo(u)r, And Comedy

As I have thought about Party Time! and other instances of hospital humor, I settled on six aspects that help explain why humans are willing—even compelled—to create jokes, black humor, and other imaginative linguistic structures that respond to the bizarre and threatening stimuli of illness, accidents, debility, and death. These are: (1) talking past taboo (including playful uses of language), (2) the power of imagery, (3) the comfort of other literary elements, in particular character and narrative, (4) attacks upon characters or ideas, (5) the themes of sex and death, and (6) throughout, the rituals that recognize the world of the sick and the world of the well and that seek their reintegration. The first three are largely literary aspects, while the second three are more thematic; clearly there are overlaps between them, and a good joke may combine several or all of them. These aspects—which will guide and organize much of the rest of this book—can be illustrated with the Party Time! ritual just described.

1. Talking Past Taboo

When a nurse says Party Time! she or he puts language to an unpleasant event about to happen, an event that "should be left unsaid" in polite society. This speech act recognizes the event and communicates to another nurse that they share the same feelings and meanings about tying up a patient. Party Time! evaluates the event through the metaphor of sex and allows the two nurses at the file cabinet to agree on their multi-layered meanings, both rational and irrational. The notion of consensual sex in the ER is, of course, a taboo subject.

Taboo (or tabu) is a Polynesian word that describes subjects that are too important or dangerous to name. These subjects vary from culture to culture and vary within a culture depending on the social setting: some topics are not mentioned at the dinner table, although they may be discussed elsewhere. Topics that are commonly taboo in polite America include the human body as it is deformed or injured, debility (including loss of memory), and death. Also, animality of humans, excrement, sex, and extreme or absurd violence. All of these are present (or implied, as in loss of sexual function) in hospital and medical settings. They are the "elephants in every room" of a hospital, unspoken subjects—with our attendant fears—that need to be addressed and somehow managed. Medical treatment is one response, of course, a discipline that is both rational and disciplined. But our minds and emotions want more, both in medical settings and in the culture at large: hospital humor attempts to satisfy our needs on emotional and instinctive levels. Medical personnel must routinely face difficult and tragic circumstances in people's lives such as car wrecks, home accidents, accidents involving tools and industrial equipment (severed fingers, a crushed hand), even a stingray that landed in a fisherman's boat and stung him severely. These suggest a world gone wrong: betrayals by our homes, machines, and nature herself. Suicide attempts and person-on-person crime are similarly disquieting. And there are reactions to drugs, both licit and illicit, alcohol, or chemicals that increasingly permeate modern life. (A trauma surgeon told me that alcohol or drugs had impaired at least half of her patients at the time of their accidents.) For other illnesses routinely seen in the ER—asthmatic attacks, diabetic crises, and heart attacks—the betrayal (if we may call it that) seems to come from within the body. No one comes to the ER for a checkup or a well-baby visit; people come because they are in pain and distress. Something has *emerged* disruptively within their lives, a sudden event clearly not expected.

Taboos often recognize the power (*mana* for Polynesians) of something. A current literary example of taboo is the villainous but mana-filled He-Who-Must-Not -Be-Named, secretly known by all to be the evil Voldemort, in J. K. Rowling's popular Harry Potter novels.

Humor is a way around taboo, so that the difficult subject can be named and, at a symbolic level, controlled. Among humorous conventions are so-called "black humor" and "sick jokes" with subject matter that is macabre, morbid, even perverse—material that society generally regards as taboo, a dark side of reality, as opposed to the happy utopias suggested by advertisements, greeting cards, theme parks, and Disney movies.

Word magic, then and now

In the ancient and folk worlds, to know the name of something—whether Jehovah or Rumpelstiltskin—was to have access to it, even control over it. This belief, called Word Magic, assumed that language captured the essence of something (see Ernst Cassirer's Chapter Four, *Language and Myth*[3]). Thus, words and phrases like "Open Sesame," "Abracadabra," or other charms and incantations made something happen at the wish of the speaker. Even today, a shaman might name an evil spirit and exorcise it from a patient in a tribe with such beliefs. Educated westerners typically don't believe in Word Magic as such; indeed for many, using the Lord's name in vain is acceptable because they do not believe the Lord will show up when called: therefore many moderns swear freely without imagined consequences. Nonetheless, we have our own secular versions of Word Magic. We dislike it intensely if our own names (or titles or addresses) are mispronounced or misspelled, a verbal attack on our identity.

Further, we take comfort from the power of other namings, for example the word or phrase that a doctor gives us as a diagnosis for an ailment or injury. While we may not consider such language absolute, it is still powerful in definition and description; we like hearing language for what's wrong with us (and I'm speaking of routine illness, not catastrophic illness), because the words suggest that the problem is now defined, the doctor knows what it is, and a conventional story of treatment can move forward. The phrase Party Time! has its own word magic, as if the phrase could control the harsh reality of tying up a patient.

For worlds that are different from ours, a literary or cinematic representation is safe and comforting. TV shows on medical subjects abound, whether fictional (*St. Elsewhere, ER, Chicago Hope, Scrubs, Crossing Jordan, House, Grey's Anatomy, Bones*) or journalistic (the Discovery Health Channel). Audiences watch safely at home with family, pets, snacks, ideal lighting and temperature, etc., happily observing gruesome material—always with the choice to look away or to turn it off. Medical caregivers are sometimes amused at these Hollywood versions, which have distortions, errors, and omissions (such as boring periods in hospitals and firehouses when little happens). During my E.M.T. training, I watched a paramedic show at a fire station with a group of firefighters; they made endless fun of the show's errors and idealistic and immediate solutions to all human dilemmas. When I told an ER nurse from another hospital that I was a volunteer in an ER, she scoffed, "If you want to shovel shit with me, just come visit *my* ER," as if the difference between my experience (a naïve volunteer in the ER) and her experience could not possibly be bridged, as if some taboos were absolute, as if I shouldn't wish to crash her own difficult but rewarding party.

Word Play, Including Puns and Euphemisms

Word play can be of many sorts, including puns, the so-called "lowest form of humor." (See Chapter Five.) Punsters enjoy playing with medical language for the fun of it and/or as a criticism of a jargon that masks reality. One particular masking is the *euphemism*, a word or phrase that makes something sound nicer than it really is, as in "patient put into restraints" instead of "tying up a real jerk."

Party Time! has its own stability and evocative power as a phrase parallel to "nap time" and "dinner time," both suggesting escape from work and responsibility. For several years beer commercials assured us that it was "Miller time." The word "party," of course, invokes birthday parties, New Year's Eve parties, and other pleasant festivities.

At a deeper level, "party" has to do with division, as in "partition" or "party to a lawsuit," an underlying structure for separation of people, which can be pleasant ("a private party") or tragic as in sickness, insanity, and death. Separation from the world of the well into the hospital world can be unpleasant or even downright terrifying, especially for patients coming to the ER because of a car wreck or an industrial accident.

Party Time!—in three neat syllables, with two crisp "t" sounds—symbolizes, in ironic and indirect fashion, qualities that humans prize: collegiality, pleasure, and freedom.

2. IMAGERY

A literary image is an appeal to the senses: a poem might mention the smell of lemons, the touch of dry leaves, the sound of a drum, or the taste of wine. The most common images, however, are visual: suggestions of size, shape, color, texture, distance from us, and so on. Compared with other mammals, humans are particularly visual in perceiving and interpreting their surroundings and their own bodies. Our interest in the opposite sex is highly visual: witness attention to physique, clothing, makeup, hair coloring, and plastic surgery. The physical mass of the body is, however, often an impediment to our freedom and our perceptions of our sexual power, especially when we are sick or injured. In Chapter Six, we will look at humorous corporeal images and their mechanical limitations, drawing on the theories of Henri Bergson's Le Rire (Laughter, 1913).[4] The power of literary images can be explained in part by their ability to represent and interpret reality. Hemingway's memorable sentence, "She was built with curves like the hull of a racing yacht" in The Sun Also Rises gives us the feeling that the character is a fast, elegant, and expensive woman—even if we don't know much about yachts' hulls. What we understand, perhaps subconsciously, are associations, suggestions, and evocations. In reading or hearing certain words, we have a parallel, visceral experience of the senses involved; we re-create images in our imaginations and personalize the meanings and emotions of the text. If the image is of something we already know, we feel pleasures of recognition. If it is foreign, we can safely domesticate or familiarize it, especially if other aspects of the text are helpful. In Ted's comment about the patient thrashing about in M-3, we can compare our known visual sense of a swimmer's backstroke with the (probably) unknown sight of a seizing patient.

In the phrase Party Time! we have not only the sarcastic image of sexual revelry between nurse and patient but also the most ironic suggestion that they are social equals who are about to spend celebrative time together, even in a busy Emergency Room. The images of the leather restraints are thus imaginatively and momentarily recast from physical restriction to many possibilities of sexual play.

3. Enclosing Unpleasant Material in Esthetic Structures

The language and imagery just mentioned are, of course, also esthetic structures, but we may turn to other, more pervasive literary structures, namely characters and stories.

Characters, including caricatures and humo(u)rous figures

Medical humor is intensely about people, because people live in bodies that may become ill and because people turn to other people for healing. The characters of medical jokes are not, however, developed characters with the depth of people we know. Rather, they are simple representations, puppets, or caricatures. In *Aspects of the Novel*, E. M. Forster suggested that literary characters could be grouped into two categories, round (or complex) and flat (or simple) and that each has uses within a novel.[5] The round figures have many motivations; these are the major characters in a novel that have the capacity to surprise us. In contrast, the flat characters have only one or two motivations, and they serve well as background figures; they are essential for a novel, since there just isn't room to make all characters round. Flat characters are generic types that we can quickly accept without worrying about their histories, relationships, or personal feelings. We might call them "caricatures," but this doesn't lessen their power, because, as types, they seem universal, characters who access our interest and belief, because we all share traits with them and because they don't have characteristics that allow us to distance ourselves from them. A Mr. or Mrs. Smith in a joke is Everyman or Everywoman; he or she represents aspects of all of us.

In this discussion, I'll use "humor" for the usual modern sense of something funny but "humour," the Middle English spelling, to refer to a specific kind of character and an ancient theory of personality. The origin of our modern word "humor" is the original Latin word "humor," or "umor," which, at base, means "liquid." (Indeed in modern biology we still refer to the vitreous and aqueous humors that fill the two chambers of the eye.) But for the ancient Greek world—Pythagoras included—the humours were fluids that pervaded the body and made it work biologically and psychologically.

Humours, sources of humor

The four classic humours are: blood, black bile, yellow bile, and phlegm, each with a corresponding temperament. Ideally, the four humours in a person should be in balance, creating a balanced temperament, but usually one is slightly on the ascendant. For example, if the humour of *blood* predominates, we have a *sanguine* character, one who is active and inclined to amorous pursuits. If blood is very out of balance, we have a Don Juan who deserves to be made fun of (humorous satire) or even cast out of society as a libidinous scapegoat. If it is *black bile*, the character is *melancholic* (*melan* meaning "black"), someone with a sad personality; jokes about this person may indeed be black humor. (See Chapter Seven for a fuller discussion.) In the ancient Greek world, these four humours related to the four elements (earth, air, water, and fire) and the four seasons of the year in a unified vision of the workings of the world and all human inhabitants.

Figure 3.1   THE FOUR HUMOURS

HUMOUR	TEMPERAMENT	ELEMENT	QUALITY	SEASON
Blood	Sanguine	Air	Wet/Hot	Spring
Yellow Bile	Choleric	Fire	Hot/Dry	Summer
Black Bile	Melancholic	Earth	Dry/Cold	Fall
Phlegm	Phlegmatic	Water	Cold/Wet	Winter

To moderns—who believe in over 100 atomic elements—the humoural view of people and the world may seem quaintly naïve; nonetheless that theory dominated medical thinking, philosophy, and literature in the West for some 2,000 years, all the way through Shakespeare, who used humour characters routinely. By contrast, germ theory—and all that it implies for asepsis, sterilization, immune responses, communicable diseases, and more—is less than 200 years old. And humour characters still appear in comic movies and cartoons in the variations of randy types (sanguine), hotheads (cholerics), sad sacks (melancholics), and couch potatoes (phlegmatics). The implied lovers of Party Time! would be sanguine characters. We have outdated phrases "to be in good humor" or "to have a good humor," meaning to be happy, but the Good Humor Trucks were famous for decades and Good Humor Ice Cream is still available.

As we have seen, another character type found in jokes is the clown, a silly or downright stupid character who can be readily abused. Happy clowns are especially useful because they don't feel pain. Like the cartoon character of Wile E. Coyote in the *Road Runner* cartoons, they are indestructible: they can be kicked from here until Sunday and come back for more. The sad clown (in the tradition of Pierrot Lunaire) is also indestructible, but he (or she) feels pain.

Another simplification of people as characters is the use of animal forms—what Jung called *theriomorphs*. This is an ancient tradition that includes Balaam's ass, mentioned eight times in the Bible, the animals of Aesop's *Fables*, and the animal characters in the medieval *fabliaux*; all these suggest continuity between humans and animals, a continuity that polite society ignores and considers taboo. We routinely speak of humans and animals as two different categories of life. Nevertheless, animal characters have long been used to represent characteristics of humans, as in the sly fox, the dumb ass, and the wise owl. Another sense of animality is sexual behavior, as in the Shakespearean phrase "the beast with two backs" (*Othello*, I.i.116-117), again often considered a taboo area in polite society. St. Francis called his body Fra Asino (Brother Ass) and asked forgiveness of it upon his deathbed for not taking better care of it. Many modern comic strips use animals, from "Pogo" to "Peanuts," from "Mutts" to "Rhymes with Orange," from "Get Fuzzy" to "Pearls before Swine," as ways of representing human behavior.

Stories and genres

Neither Ted's backstroker nor the implied Party Time! patient offer much of a story; they are both images of patients in difficulty. A somewhat abstract and implied story, however, is a version of the Night Sea Journey, with the basic structure of stasis/chaos/stasis; in both cases caregivers seek to return the patient to the stasis of health. This is a classic story form: thousands of TV shows follow this pattern, especially cop shows: normalcy/crime/resolution. In the medical world, we have two intensifications: (1) the primary conflict resides, not on a city street, but in the *body* of a human being, and (2) there are two overlapping categories of people, the world of the sick and the world of the well. Although we all live on the same planet, the differences in consciousness of being well or sick (and I mean more than colds or twisted ankles) are profound. Anyone who experiences a life-threatening illness—whether as a patient, a family member, or a friend—knows about these two worlds and deeply wishes, at a primal level, for the patient's departure from the world of the sick and return to the world of the well.

In stories with medical subjects, there are the usual, major genres: plays (Molière's *Le medecin malgre lui*), novels (Samuel Shem's *The House of God*), and short stories (Steve Martin's "Artist Lost to Zoloft" in *Pure Drivel*.[6] We also find a series of subgenres in oral humor: riddles, one-liners, catch phrases, short stories, shaggy dog stories, knock knock jokes, spoonerisms, and so on, conventions that give order and shape our expectations.

Myth

One source of stories is the realm of myths (indeed the Greek word means "story"). Post-enlightenment moderns often speak of myths as stories that are not true ("the moon is made of green cheese"), but all cultures have their mythic stories of heroes and their victories that exemplify cultural values—for example, sacred scriptures, epic poems, even the legend of George Washington and the cherry tree. Such stories are told and retold, literary rituals that entertain us, inform us, and shape our values. The Night Sea Journey is a classic mythic form.

4. Attacks on Characters, Institutions, and Ideas

Sigmund Freud carefully laid out the notion of attack in humor in his *Jokes and Their Relation to the Unconscious (Der Witze und seine Beziehung zum Unbewussen,* 1905).[7] The German *Witze* translated as "jokes" is a bit misleading, since witty comments (and especially attacking ones) were also part of his concern. Writing in repressive Vienna over a century ago, Freud found that much ironic or sarcastic humor was a veiled attack. Today the humor is often more direct, including sarcastic comments we call "cuts," "slams," or "digs" and numerous jokes that attack insurance companies, HMOs, hospitals, and doctors, specifically their position, power, or wealth (see Chapter Eight). Freud's notion of attack also includes rejection of characters as exiled scapegoats. In Party Time! the hypothetic sybarites of nurse and patient are clearly preposterous; we simultaneously mention them and cast them aside as inappropriate. Even Ted's backstroker is a substitution for the troubling patient, who is shunted aside in our minds in favor of a more athletic "person."

5. Themes of Aging and Death (even Sex)

It is hardly news to a culture with Puritan and Enlightenment roots that its underbelly includes two taboo subjects, death and sex. Comedy cheerfully and relentlessly exposes, manipulates, and celebrates both of them.

America is a culture that is death-aversive. We create structures to hide the dead from us, for example, the ban on photographs of flag-draped caskets carrying US soldiers killed in Iraq. (This policy was rescinded by the Obama administration on the advice of military families and leaders in February of 2009.) Serious injuries, whether physical or mental are also troubling. As US military personnel return from Iraq and

only country where death is an option

Afghanistan with grievous injuries, our society struggles to understand the impact. For several years government reports of these wounded downplayed their numbers and the severity of injuries. One factor in bringing media attention to them was the wounding of ABC newsman Bob Woodruff, who reported on injured soldiers as a person who is "one of us." Woodruff entered the dark world of war and returned to tell not only his story, but the story of others as well.

We routinely remove the dead from the hospital in cloaked gurneys to take them to the mortuary, where they are often costumed and made up as if still alive. If there is no viewing, the dead are hidden in a large casket (no one says "coffin" anymore). Either way, they are typically embalmed as if to make them permanent, and then, "buried" in a concrete vault (therefore not touching the earth) or burned in a crematory, leaving only fragments of the largest vertebrae and hip bones (euphemistically, the "ashes").

Advertisements, movies, and other blandishments of the "youth culture" make clear that *to be young is good* and *to be old is bad*. And to be dead is even worse. Young people, the ads tell us, play volleyball on the beach in tiny bathing suits, ready to mate and procreate at the drop of a hat. Old people—well, they have the "duty to die," as former Colorado governor Richard Lamm famously put it.

Ted's patient backstroking in his bed is, socially speaking, dead. His non-purposeful flailing portrays a tragedy—however temporary—in his life: out of control physiologically and mentally, he is sexually incompetent and not a potential progenitor. He cannot function normally as he would like and as society requires. Left in this state, he might recover, but he might also expire. It is the job of Ted, the doctors, the lab technicians, and everybody else involved in his care to bring him back to a social life without regard to cost, effort, or inconvenience to other potential patients in the waiting room. (Such patients may be nearby, perhaps on the other side of one wall, but their world of unattended sickness is miles away from a world of the sick who have been taken into medical care.)

In the dynamics of Party Time!, the out-of-control patient is socially dysfunctional. He or she cannot do activities of daily life (ADL in the occupational therapist's designation), hold a job, or act as a sexually powerful person—society's underlying, relentless demand—to create a new generation. If the patient is suffering seizures (another form of restraint), he or she is in a limbo, a liminal state between function and nonfunction (again suggestive of death), and the hospital staff is empowered and required to bring him or her back by all means possible. In terms of the humours, the *phlegmatic* or inert person should become, once again, a *sanguine* or amorous person.

6. RITUALS THAT RECOGNIZE THE WORLDS OF THE WELL AND OF THE SICK

It is a short jump to our final dynamic, the sense of rituals: the repeated, symbolic actions that represent normative values for a culture or subculture.

Let's start with the simple exchange of jokes, perhaps at a water cooler, a copy machine, or a lunch date of peers. I remember a colleague who always had a joke. Indeed I felt that I needed to have one too, just to keep up my end of the conversation. Wherever we met at work, he'd tell his and I'd tell mine, and we'd both go away happy. Why was this? The jokes themselves were usually at least moderately funny, but perhaps more important was the fact that we had had an exchange that went according to tacitly agreed expectations. We laughed at each other's care in remembering a joke, each other's skill in presenting it, and we had shared the basic structures of the joke: introduction, build up, and punch line, with the resultant shared laughter. Since we were careful not to speak about our work, we also met as multivalent humans, not as employees controlled by an institution. As we joked, we proclaimed our independence: our citizenship in the creative freedom of the Green World. (I also remember another colleague who would expect generous laughter from his listeners but would condescendingly grant only small chuckles for anyone else's jokes; apparently he wished to be perceived as "wittier than thou.")

The Party Time! participants share a practiced phrase that helps them define and keep alive their values concerning the sick and the well. They constitute a small comic community that uses code to validate their work. The nurse visiting the restraint drawer with mixed emotions gains support from the other nurses who offer the ritual phrase. Outsiders hearing this phrase might well find it inappropriate. (More on appropriateness in Chapter Twelve.)

We've spoken about "cheering up" patients. The word "cheer" has an interesting history, going back to Anglo-Norman "chere" meaning "face" or "expression" (from Latin *cara*, from Greek *kara*, meaning "head"), all suggesting "mood, as shown in the face" (*Encarta World English Dictionary*, 1999). Thus there are two important aspects, the positive mood of cheerfulness and means of expression (of face, of voice, of gesture) that communicate this mood socially to others. We think of the elaborate rituals of cheerleaders and, more generally, the uplifting behaviors of cheerful people. We'll say more about smiles in Chapter Four.

IN SUMMARY

Entering the hospital world is usually a stressful event, especially for patients in an ER. To enter the world of the sick is to leave the world of the well, to be cut off, to lose comfortable aspects of daily living and various symbols of our freedom and power: we become separated from people and things we love. When leather restraints further separate us, we are further removed, even within the world of the sick. Such separations are tragic, and our instincts (whether we are sick or well) yearn for comic restorations to health and social relationships.

We said a moment ago that the image of the nurse and patient as sexual libertines was rejected by sarcastic humor. At a mythic level, however, we could consider that the phrase Party Time! invokes a fantasy of festive wellness that might allow patient and caregiver to make love, and who's to say who would tie up whom first? In this mythos, all persons are well and capable of absolute freedom (symbolized in sexual activity), in an archetypal wedding of minds and bodies. This is the ultimate sense of comedy, that all are married to all throughout all time and space. One such version is the Christian mythos, the wedding feast of the Lamb in the New Jerusalem of Heaven.

Before this joyous apocalypse, however, we must live within a series of all too realistic confines. We live in bodies that are very human; they get sick and injured, and they have losses as we age. We rely on doctors, nurses, hospitals, HMOs and other aspects of the US healthcare "system," people and structures that are sometimes error-prone, sometimes demeaning, and always limited in their power. We use language that is powerful in some ways, but ambiguous and misleading in other ways. We live with people who are sometimes boorish, greedy, arrogant, and/or condescending. We live in a society that has some strange, even neurotic ideas about sex and death and that often deals with these by silence reinforced by taboo. In this strange world, we sometimes feel an urge to escape, to rebel and claim our freedom through humor. Sometimes the joker is the professional clown or comedian who comes to us through mass media. Sometimes the joker is someone we know who enjoys making us laugh. Sometimes the jokers are any or all of us, especially when we feel an antic urge to laugh in the face of many of these absurdities, including that, sooner or later, our bodies become injured or sick and, sooner or later, we will all die. Until that day, however, we have the freedom to tell jokes on just about any topic we choose.

A FORTY-YEAR OLD JOKE

Decades ago, the following joke made the rounds.

CAN SAMMY COME OUT?

A group of children are on the porch of the Nelsons' house. One rings the doorbell. When Mrs. Nelson answers, he says, "We're going to play softball. Can Sammy come out and play with us?"

Mrs. Nelson replies, "Well, Sammy doesn't have any arms or legs. So I don't think that would work out very well."

The child thinks a moment, then says, "Well, could he come out and be third base?"

At the time, such jokes were called "sick jokes," nominally because they dealt with human defects in body or mind, but even more, I think, because they broke norms of polite behavior which didn't mention disabilities such as Sammy's, much less make a joke about such a demeaning usage of him. By calling such a joke "sick," some audiences could both enjoy it as a joke but reject it as an unhealthy aberration from social norms, while other audiences would reject it entirely as impolite in the extreme. (It is hard to imagine a parent of a drastically deformed child—a thalidomide baby, for example—finding this joke funny.)

And yet, like the Party Time! example, Can Sammy Come Out? allows us to put into language one of our deepest fears, that our children might be deformed and therefore isolated from society. Like the patient tied up in an Emergency Room, Sammy is imprisoned in a body that can't run, walk, swing a bat, or play outside in the Green World of softball with other children. In the joke, he's reduced to a body useful only for being third base. Although Party Time! may seem odd to us, that example of clinical humor has parallels in the oral tradition of jokes such as this one. Such jokes also give voice to some of our deepest fears and hopes and, at the same time, give us ways of re-evaluating emotionally difficult subjects.

Party Time! was a kind of street theater, an improvised routine that the "actors" shared and acted out. In my description, I wrote down not only the bare script but also a speculative account of the psychodynamics behind it. On the other hand, Can Sammy Come Out?, as written out above, is exactly a script, but with none of the theater: no one at a water cooler or copy machine telling the story with gestures and eye contact, and no shared laughter between teller and listeners. But in both forms of comedy we have people dealing with troublesome (and often taboo) aspects of how we live in our bodies and how we relate to each other, especially if there is a sick or deformed person involved. And jokes about such medical topics—whether told out loud or read on email or on websites—are both diverse and numerous.

What do we find if we take the six aspects mentioned above and apply them to Can Sammy Come Out?

Talking past taboo. The joke breaks taboo by speaking of deformity in children and also breaks social norms by demeaning a deformed child.

Imagery. First we picture a child without arms or legs as an invalid ("not valid") at home; second we picture him in the ludicrous position as third base on a baseball diamond.

Esthetic structures. Character: all the speaking characters are undifferentiated types with little personality. Mrs. Nelson is guarded and careful in what she says. The child spokesman is either very naïve or perhaps even evil, but we can't tell. The off-stage Sammy is a *phlegmatic* type, apparently taking no action in life. The story is a classic joke format, with a situation, a build-up, and a quick punch line that diverges from normal social discourse. We have a parody of a familiar negotiation format with a question, a denial, and a second question, although this last question is, of course, absurd.

Freudian attack. Sammy is demeaned for being outside the social norms of the children, in physical appearance and ability. The joke allows us to confirm our dislike for such limitations. At the same time, the spokesman for the group of children can be considered an evil person, one whom we reject through our laughter.

Rituals that recognize the communities of the well and the sick. The children on the porch are well and active; they ask if Sammy can join them. When Mrs. Nelson says no, Sammy becomes a scapegoat, someone rejected because he doesn't fit. When the child asks about third base, we are caught between two moods, an earnest request that Sammy join in the fun versus the wildly inappropriate image of him as third base. If we find the joke funny, we laugh at this tension, and even at the off-stage Sammy, consigning him (cruelly) to the eternal realm of the sick. We congratulate ourselves that we are not part of this world and go on about our business—unless, of course, we consider the joke to be loathsome and reject it entirely as truly being "sick."

Party Time! and Can Sammy Come Out? have similarities and seem to work well with the six aspects discussed so far. The former developed in a specific ER culture while the other is a joke from the wider popular culture, but both examples are ironic, even sarcastic humor that deals with difficult subjects of restrictions on human freedom. Both employ image, mood, and character in order to create an acceptance and even control of taboo subject matter.

In the next chapter, we will compare these two examples to the gentler, more comforting humor we saw in Vonnie the hospital clown.

Chapter Four

From Comforting Clowns to Ironic Jokers

The Many Kinds and Purposes of Comedy

THE COMIC WORK of Vonnie the hospital clown and the raucous humor of Party Time! seem so far apart that finding commonalities may seem unlikely, if not impossible. The two exhibits are quite dissimilar in the images overlaid on a sickroom: a circus clown who would appear before a large crowd versus an imagined couple practicing erotic bondage in private. Further, the two exhibits are widely dissimilar in mood, the first gently cheerful and upbeat, the second wildly ironic, even sarcastic. Nevertheless, there are continuities between these two extremes: they both deal with unhealth, promote positive changes in emotions, create a Green World of comedy within the gray world of the hospital, and establish and sustain comic communities.

In this chapter, I'd like to discuss our two extremes of humor so that (1) we can see how they can illuminate each other, (2) we may explore the more specific roles of clown and joker, and (3) we may discuss the interacting qualities of comfort and irony.

A CLOWNISH VIEW OF THE PARTY TIME! PEOPLE

If we take the four pervasive qualities identified in Vonnie's hospital clowning, we can pose them as questions to the Party Time! event.

Is There a Comic Community? When nurses exchange the ritual phrase Party Time! at the file cabinet with the drawer of restraints, they make up a small comic community, one which does not include patients, relatives, administrators, or the public at large. The nurses use this phrase as code, shorthand for values they share: *yes, we are nurses; we do all sorts of distasteful duties for every kind of patient, even the most unruly, dirty, or violent patient.* At the same time, there is another, deeper message that includes nurses in a universal group of healthy human beings: *we affirm that we are healthy, sexually alive persons who celebrate the possibilities of erotic freedom.* Even while dealing with a sickest of humans, nurses can comically affirm sexuality as a fixed point, like magnetic north.

Are There Modulations of Desire? I didn't interview nurses about this ritual, so I don't know how they'd answer this question. Even if I had discussed it with them, they might not have been conscious of the dynamics of emotion involved. What follows, therefore, is my speculative interpretation. In the Party Time! phrase, the nurses deal with their emotions that may include any or all of the following: (A) distaste, pity, fear, sadness, scorn, even loneliness, and they seek to awaken such emotions as (B) resolve, understanding, obligation, and acceptance. (We might consider this shift from A to B a telescoped form of Elisabeth Kübler-Ross's five stages of grief, from denial all the way to acceptance.) My reading is that the nurses feel the emotional support of their joking colleagues: *this is my job, and I can do it, because we nurses maintain our social solidarity even in the face of the absurd.*

Are There Links to the Green Past? This is perhaps the clearest of the four qualities; the Party Time! formula suggests that: *we nurses are alive, we are healthy, and one marker of our health is sexual energy and viability that might, if we chose, be expressed in an erotic act of bondage.* Furthermore, not only might such sexuality be expressed in the past or future outside of the hospital, it might—outrageously—be expressed right here in the ER—during work!

Are There Changes in Qualities of Space? Restraining a patient is an extreme limitation of spatial freedom—a symbol for the more general senses of imprisonment of being sick, being in an emergency room, and being out of control, a danger to self and others. The Party Time! joke creates the imaginative hypothesis that the spatial limitations of restraints could be redefined to allow for erotic pleasure in a social relationship of consent, so that the very gray world of the ER is suddenly and boisterously re-imagined as vividly Green.

I conclude that the four qualities we found in Vonnie's work are applicable to the Party Time! exhibit.

WHY SEX?

As I gathered material in medical settings and in the world of jokes, I was surprised by how often there were sexual references. Why would this be so? I think there are several reasons. First, there's a basic affirmation of sex, which can be most pleasurable, an activity of intimacy and love, and a fulfillment of longing and desire. These values are deep, on the primal level of instinct; they provide energy, interest, and excitement to comedy.

Second, there's a wider sense of generativity and creativity that often doesn't fit with the mundane, 9-to-5, gotta-make-money rat race. Sexual activity (even reckless abandon!) is not something to be mentioned in so-called "polite society," which seems to assume that ecstatic sexual bliss is impossible to find or that it can only be illicit or that, in any case, we certainly don't deserve it. Given attitudes of repression and denial, joking references to sex can affirm our interest in and desire for sex as a path to adventure, variety, and freedom.

Third, there's energy (even rebellion) in breaking taboos that repress or ignore sex, especially in a culture with Puritan roots. In contemporary America, there are forces that consider sex as "something nice people don't talk about"; such forces may include religion, intellectualism, academia, professionalism, elitism, and asceticism. If sex is to be talked about at all, it would be only in specific situations such as formal writing or a smaller, intimate setting, where all participants agree on the linguistic norms. When jokers use sexual themes and imagery, they stretch language away from ordinary polite usage and suggest an intimacy between speaker and audience, an intimacy that may or may not be welcome to listeners.

A further complication is that people may have two sets of values regarding taboo material, one for public discourse and another for private discourse. Public discourse is more formal, in part because the sensitivities of all persons in the audience cannot be known. A comedian who deals in "blue material" would not be welcome at many gatherings, although he or she might be well accepted at a comedy club, where the audience comes voluntarily, knowing in advance the sort of humor to be presented.

Furthermore there's a "backstage" effect: actors and musicians often share wild-and-crazy (to borrow Steve Martin's phrase) humor among themselves, in endless rehearsals, in waiting backstage, and after performances, but while onstage in front of an audience, they fit the exact decorum required of them. Backstage, they are a comic community that needs humor to relieve tension, to bond the members, to cope with stress, to keep creative juices flowing. Genevieve Parsons et al. discuss the dynamics of "backstage" speech and the differences of "insiders" and "outsiders" when humor and slang are used in medical settings, often making medical students uncomfortable.[1] The notion of "backstage" becomes greatly compromised, however, when electronic media are involved. Students may think they are sharing jokes only with each other, when in fact the whole cyber world can listen. In a posting to the Literature and Medicine listserve sponsored by the American Society of Bioethics and Humanities, physician and bioethicist Jay Baruch wrote, "I'm amazed how stunningly smart students don't always grasp the implications of the blogging and social networking activities. They all sat up, however, when I revealed how admissions committees, residency directors, and potential employers might Google them when considering their applications for education and job opportunities."[2] He cited three recent discussions that raise ethical issues concerning material, humorous or not, placed on social networks.[3]

In each of these three reasons—primal pleasure, creativity, and breaking taboo—we find that sex is often considered good, vital, perhaps even utopian. It is a basic feature of the Green World, a place of pleasure, intimacy, love, and generation of children. It has the metaphoric status of solid footing. But sexual references are not always good, welcome, or appropriate. In a few pages, we'll return to the wider topic of appropriateness.

A Party Time!-Ish View Of Vonnie

We may test Vonnie's clowning against the six aspects identified in our discussion of Party Time!

Talking past taboo? There's not much to report here beside a hint at bowel regularity, mention of the off-stage doctor who fell down, plus a comment about the difficulties in grooming, and the mild attacks on hospital food and gowns. Vonnie, as a hospital clown, generally sticks to safe subjects.

Imagery? Vonnie herself is the dominant and powerful image; she can be recognized a hundred feet away, and all her visual props deepen and reinforce her image as a clown. Vonnie refers to images of patients (hair, gown) as part of her conversation, making clear that she sees and accepts them even in their hospitalized state. She responds *imaginatively* to the image of a patient who can't reach to scratch her legs.

Esthetic structures? Vonnie is a known, traditional character, a figure of joy and sociability, much like Ronald McDonald or Patch Adams, the real-life hospital clown. For all such clowns, the humour is *sanguine*, as in vital blood, and the color red figures prominently in Vonnie's makeup. Thus she brings sanguine energy into the phlegmatic space of the hospital.

For story, we don't find much. Vonnie works from a brief scenario: *knock at the door; if invited, enter; observe and listen; make jokes accordingly; offer gifts; say goodbye and depart.* Within this scheme she is free to offer her version of improv comedy—in contrast to joke tellers who tell jokes in a classic joke format. Her esthetic is to think on her feet, working from patients' visual cues and what they say to her.

Freudian attack? Not a lot, except for the comments about hospital food and gowns. Perhaps the doctor who fell down with a bloody nose provides patients with a symbolic target for attack, a way of releasing anger, but this would be at an unconscious level, and patients would, furthermore, differ widely in responses. If attack there is, it's a gentle rebellion, a sweet subversion of hospital space to clowning and cheerful foolishness.

Themes of aging and death? Not much. Vonnie acknowledges the patients' illnesses, especially if they mention them, and she emphasizes their progress in healing, but she does not make jokes about these two topics. Death remains an invisible elephant in the room, fully cloaked by taboo.

Communities of the well and the sick? Vonnie ritually brings the known and festive world of the circus into the uncertain, depressing, and gray world of the hospital. Vonnie draws into her comic community not only patients, but relatives, visitors, nurses, and me, a visiting observer. She gives her performance to complete strangers, hands out candy to passers-by, and makes conversation possible between people who don't know each other. She is a magnet, a catalyst who creates ad hoc communities quickly. These small communities echo a distant but archetypal community of people attending a circus, people who are "children of all ages," in the ringmaster's traditional phrase. The circus itself is a mythic image of wellness, where the performers tame wild animals, acrobats defy gravity, and clowns fall down and rise up. For the moment, sickness and mortality are forgotten, and jovial wellness reigns supreme.

The six aspects of the Party Time! exhibit help illuminate some of the aspects of Vonnie's work by what they have in common and how they differ. They diverge, of course, in the sharpness of criticism of unpleasant subjects, and the kind and intensity of mood. One excludes patients while the other includes them. What they have in common is the ritual affirmation of the basic solidarity and collegiality of persons through references to the past, specifically the pleasant experiences of the circus and erotic activity. These are controlling metaphors, comparisons with strong images and emotional content, so that a participant can imagine himself or herself pleasurably transported to a world that is wonderfully Green.

THE ROLES OF CLOWNS AND JOKERS

Let us turn to our two central character types, clowns and jokers, to see what they have in common and where they diverge. In common parlance, the terms overlap. Perhaps all of us as youngsters were admonished to "stop clowning around," when we thought we were just joking. For our purposes here, I'll suggest that "joker" is the larger term and "clown" is a specialized subset, a particular tradition within the larger realm of joking. Indeed, given that all humans make jokes, we can consider it a universal activity of people, even a marker of humanity. As Rabelais put it in his Prologue to *Gargantua*, "to laugh is natural to man" ("rire est le propre de l'homme"). Other mammals (dogs, cats, chimps) also enjoy jokes of rudimentary sorts, but the range of human joking is magnificently wide, from stand-up comics to humorous email messages, from outrageous practical jokes to sitcoms on TV, from playing peek-a-boo with babies to sophisticated improv comedy, from puns to sleight-of-hand tricks, from Halloween costumes to waggish commentary, from satire to parody to travesty. I'll use the term joker in the widest sense of anyone who makes jokes, whether wild and crazy at one extreme—or, at the other extreme, gentle.

In the realm of the most gentle, we can mention "smilers," perhaps the subtlest form of humor, but nonetheless sometimes very powerful. A woman told me of her experience in a hospital: "I was in a terrible auto accident that nearly killed me. I was in bed, considering that death was imminent and preparing myself for that event. Unexpectedly, a Jamaican orderly (or janitor—I never knew what his role was) took my two hands in his and smiled broadly at me. He said nothing, but I felt that this moment was the turning point in my healing." Buddhist monk Thich Nhat Hahn has written about smiles: "Smiling means that we are ourselves, that we have sovereignty over ourselves, that we are not drowned into forgetfulness. This kind of smile can be seen on the faces of Buddhas and Bodhisattvas." He calls smiling "the most basic

FIGURE 4.1: JOKERS, CLOWNS, AND SMILERS: RANGES OF HUMOR

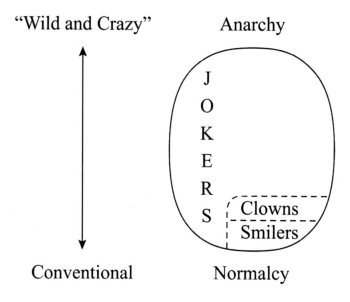

kind of peace work."[4] Indicating friendly intentions, smiles can be useful and positive in many settings, including health-related ones. In Figure 4.1, the dotted lines suggest that the categories aren't strict but fluid, with overlaps.

THE ROLE OF INTENTION

The concept of intention may seem hopelessly vague and/or subjective. Indeed, Lynne McTaggart (in her serious book *The Intention Experiment*) warns that for some, "Intention has become the latest new age buzzword."[5] Nonetheless, she writes some three hundred pages (including fifty pages of notes and bibliography) about scientific investigations of intention, including mind-body interactions, distant healing, martial artists, healers, and group mind events. Many of the concepts are beyond standard Western thought and education, although various Eastern and mystical traditions have their own versions and uses (and have had these for centuries, even millennia). Sports psychology is now one of the more widely known practical applications, although numerous popular accounts seek to make intention a servant of success, happiness, even wealth (see, for example, Wayne W. Dyer, *The Power of Intention.*[6]) Drawing on quantum physics, McTaggart (and others) speak of coherence and synchrony within persons and entrainment and entanglement between persons, often beyond the realm of the conscious mind. I believe this line of inquiry will eventually tell us more about how comedy and humor work and why they are powerful. For now, I'll suggest that the intentions of a joke teller (to entertain, to give pleasure, to practice a known art form) are perceived by a listener who may choose whether to join the ritual; if the listener participates, it's with an intention to pay attention, to enjoy the narrative in its traditional form plus the variations, and to laugh with the teller and any others, all of whom form an intentional comic community. In a health-care setting, these shared intentions can be very powerful.

JOKING AS A PERVASIVE AND CENTRAL HUMAN ACTIVITY

Humans are a species enamored with joking. We may consider three reasons jokes are central to human existence: (1) joking constitutes a claim to freedom, (2) joking gives us a sense of agency and control, and (3) joking gives us pleasure. Furthermore, these three functions are all socially sanctioned by tradition and daily practice. If a coworker at the copy machine or water cooler says, "Say, did you hear the one about the doctor?" we know what to expect, and we're usually glad to delay any job in order to hear a joke in the company of a friendly person.

1. Joking Constitutes a Claim to Freedom

Joking is an opposite of the world of duty, function, calculation, and seriousness, cultural norms that may seem limiting. Making jokes reminds us of children who can follow their desires more or less freely; we speak of "kidding around," that is, acting like kids (i. e., frolicsome goats). The joker in the card deck can mean whatever a game decides; he's an open field. In joking we explore the possible; an elaborate joke can be fantastic, unconstrained by physics and other natural laws. If politics is the "art of the possible," joking is the art of the possible *and* the impossible, making crazy things plausible, at least for the comic moment. Whether we're telling a joke or hearing one, we are, for that time, in a realm of freedom. This isn't total anarchy because verbal jokes have traditional structures. The limerick, for example, has specific structures for meter and rhyme, into which ingenious language is fitted.

Johan Huizinga describes three essentials of the human race: *Homo sapiens* (wise human), *Homo faber* (the making or crafting human) and *Homo ludens* (the playing human).[7] He sees play in all its attributes as nonrational but essential to our deepest nature, and nonreducible to other terms: "All the terms in this loosely connected group of ideas—play, laughter, folly, wish, jest, joke, the comic, etc.—share the characteristic which we had to attribute to play, namely, that of resisting any attempt to reduce it to other terms. Their rationale and their mutual relationships must lie in a very deep layer of our mental being" (*Homo Ludens*, p. 6). Huizinga's formulation about play fully applies to much of joking, in particularly its freedom within arbitrary limits:

> It is an activity which proceeds within certain limits of time and space, in a visible order, according to rules freely accepted, and outside the sphere of necessity or material utility. The play-mood is one of rapture and enthusiasm, and is sacred or festive in accordance with the occasion. A feeling of exaltation and tension accompanies the acting, mirth and relaxation follow (p. 132).

We may be reluctant to go to a hospital to visit a seriously ill friend, but we have little reluctance to tell or hear a joke about hospitals because of its esthetic safety. If, however, the joke is satiric or sarcastic, Huizinga's value-free argument does not apply because comedy that criticizes people, ideas, and institutions does indeed have utility, purpose, and clear morals.

2. Joking Gives Us Feelings of Agency and Control

We make jokes because they give us the feeling—however temporary or illusory—of agency and control. Agency means that we are capable of taking action, doing things, as opposed to being passive victims. When we are injured or sick, making jokes is a way of validating that we still have power. When he was shot, President Reagan was reported to have cracked jokes in the ER of George Washington University Hospital. Sick people often joke about their limitations, a kind of vengeance on the one hand, but also a claim of verbal control in the tradition of Word Magic discussed earlier.

Furthermore, to tell a joke is to take the spotlight, to perform for an audience. In joking we entertain, giving something to an audience. (Compulsive jokers, however, are often not welcome, in part because they seek to have too much control over social settings.) A person telling a joke displays control of the art form in using characters, plots, climactic pacing, and a punch line. If the subject matter is medical, teller and hearer have a sense of control over that topic.

3. Joking Gives Us Pleasure

Whether we consciously sense freedom or control, we clearly sense pleasure. When the circumstances are right, joking is fun, jolly, pleasurable—and pleasure is one of the most basic of all human motivators. If we hear a joke and laugh, we're happy. If we tell a joke and people laugh, we're happy. Whether it's two people laughing or an audience of three hundred people, there is a social solidarity in shared laughter that is most pleasurable: our values are affirmed, and we enjoy the solidarity of belonging to the group. The pleasures of hilarity are important to us. We watch comic TV shows and go to comic movies; we visit comedy clubs and go to the circus; we tell jokes, we make playful remarks and puns, and we play with each other through many forms of humor, all for the fun of it.

A counter-example may occur if we come upon a TV show in the middle of a stand-up routine. Suddenly we see an audience laughing like hyenas. The camera switches back to the comedian, and we listen a moment, puzzled that s/he doesn't seem funny at all. Why is this? Evidently, we don't "have her/his wave length," we are not part of the group hysteria, and, clearly, we are not part of that particular comic community in the auditorium that night. We may wonder, "How much have these people had to drink?" or muse: "I guess you had to have *been there.*" Humor works when comic moods and expectations have been established and it often also intensifies during the event as people join in psychologically and physically (laughing, clapping, whooping). There are also instances of unexpected comic humor: sometimes these work, if an audience can change moods quickly, but often they do not.

JOKING, THE DARK SIDE

Jokers can be gadflies, goads, or agents provocateurs. Jokers can have positive, neutral, or negative influences, depending on their level of ferocity and on the audience hearing them, but all of them subvert conventions of logic and order. A practical joke can be harmless, but a computer hack might cost a company millions of dollars. Political satirists from Art Buchwald to Andy Borowitz are outgrowths of the court jester, who could poke or prod royalty, often with moral intention. The fool in *King Lear* is a joker who speaks the truth, even through riddles. On the other hand, the Joker in the Batman comics and movies is an arch-villain, a sociopath who commits brutal crimes; he lives in furthest margins of the ironic, gray world, the realm of frightening anarchy; his intention appears to be a combination of evil and chaos. Today, stand-up comics work alone, and can say anything they like, whether it's insulting, racist, sexist, or obscene. So-called "Shock Jocks" on radio and TV are similar, although they can get into trouble with listening audiences, their bosses, their commercial sponsors, or the Federal Communications Commission.

If the target of attacking humor hears it directly, there may be tragic implications. Many of us remember a lesson in intention from elementary school something like this: "Now children, are we actually laughing *with* little Johnnie or are we laughing *at* him?" I remember being jolted by this formulation because I understood that I myself might be laughed at and become a third-grade scapegoat. A dark side of joking is the realm of satire, sarcasm, and derision—attacks on persons, ideals, or institutions. In the case of persons, the humor can have the aim of shunning or expulsion from a social group, a form of tragedy in Frye's terms. (Recently there's been much discussion of bullying in schools, another instance of social rejection.) Our legal system has provisions for libel and slander to protect persons from defaming language that might come from a malign joker. This protection is not absolute, however, and many people have felt the pain of ridicule without any legal recourse. We may hopefully assert that "Sticks and stones will break my bones, but names will never hurt me," but we know that this often is not true, because names, innuendoes, allegations, and direct verbal attacks can hurt people personally, socially, politically, even professionally and financially. Finally, joking within some communities that seems fine to those participants may seem inappropriate or unethical by observers from other communities. Every few years a public figure gets into trouble when remarks meant for a small audience are broadcast widely through an open microphone.

Issues of appropriate humor have been raised for medical education. In an article "Making Fun of Patients: Medical Students' Perceptions and Use of Derogatory and Cynical Humor in Clinical Settings," Delese Wear, et al., argue that jokes about patients can be part of an "ethical erosion" in medical students, and that such humor is by and large inappropriate and should be discouraged by medical educators.[8] The article discusses disparaging comments about obese patients, drug users, and other patients who do not follow good health habits. (Because the patients involved did not hear these comments, direct satiric attack is not at issue.) The students surveyed agree that some subjects (cancer in children, for example) are "off limits," which suggests some ethical concern. Some inappropriate humor comes from attending physicians or residents, while the lower-in-status medical students wonder about ethical norms of humorous speech about patients and, ethically enough, find some humor by persons in authority to be inappropriate. The article's emphasis on "derogatory" and "cynical" humor, furthermore, seems to allow for other humors that are ironic but not attacking and even humors that actually affirm the patient. My experience with first-year medical students in the anatomy lab was that there was plenty of humor, that it was not demeaning of the cadavers, and that it was within a comic community that shared, more or less, the same positive norms (see *First Cut: A Season in the Human Anatomy Lab*, especially pp. 127, 164, 192-93, 235).[9]

DILEMMAS OF APPROPRIATENESS

While comedy can have several benefits, it can cause problems or be harmful when conditions are not right. Here is a brief list of factors that may make humor inappropriate:

1. Stringency. Especially in medicine, when time pressure and seriousness of tasks (saving a life, for example) are important, comedy can distract, perhaps even cause errors.

2. Seriousness. When a mood is traditionally serious (as in a religious service), comedy doesn't fit.

3. Absolute taboos. In social groups where certain topics are taboo, comedy breaking those taboos would be inappropriate.

4. Partial or conditional taboos. Jokers or comedians may have to "test the waters" or even ask whether some topics are admissible for humor.

5. Attacking humor that demeans subgroups, for example sexist or racist humor. Other all-to-easy targets in medicine include patients who are obese, damaged by tobacco, liquor, or illicit drugs, or have done violence to themselves. Healthy persons wishing to distance themselves from patients who are mentally ill have made jokes about the "short buses" that transport such children.

6. Situations of social inequality. Persons in power may assume their sort of humor has universal appeal. I recall a physician bioethicist discussing M&M confer-

Too dark to operate

ences at his hospital. (A Morbidity and Mortality conference is, essentially, a discussion of "did we do anything wrong?" and, if so, "how can we avoid that in the future?") He said that there was often extreme humor, and that he considered such humor to be healthy for that specific group, allowing the participants to deal with emotions of failure, loss, and tragedy and to have, even in depressing situations, some sense of play, creativity, and affirmation of common purpose. When, however, there were visitors such as medical students, he became worried that they might perceive such humor as disrespectful and cynical. A mixed group may or may not work as a comic community.

7. Showboating. The word "appropriate" can also be a verb meaning "acquire." A loudmouth joker may appropriate time, space, and attention through excessive joking, distracting others from their thoughts, actions, and/or common purpose. He or she can also damage group spirit and process by unrelenting sarcasm.

Our title "Clowns and Jokers Can Heal Us" is perhaps too brief and too simple. More accurately, it might read, "Clowns and Jokers Can, in Some Circumstances, Be a Resource for Healing, but They Need to Be Careful and Considerate."

Jokes As Literary Structures And Mental Processes

Dictionaries such as Oxford and Encarta tell us that the word *joke* has its origin in the Latin *jocus* which means *jest* or *wordplay*. (It's good to know that joking goes back at least that far and that the Romans, all orderly and governmental, had a sense of humor.) Jokes are an important strand in the oral tradition, something we recognize immediately, whether from a politician opening a speech with a joke, a comedian starting a routine, or any group of people starting to tell jokes. Once cued that a joke is coming, we expect certain moods, conventional characters, evocative language, a narrative building to a punch line, and the chance to join others in laughter.

In this discussion, I'm focusing on jokes as verbal structures (and not practical jokes, musical jokes, or visual jokes such as optical illusions). Literary jokes include formal conventions such as puns, riddles, limericks, spoonerisms, and shaggy dog stories.[10] Such forms give structure and shape to our expectations. We readily recognize satires and parodies. The content, of course, can range widely from gentle humor to ferocious sarcasm. Jokes depend on the basic elements of language, character, and narrative. The language often uses odd formulations (puns and other plays on words) and sometimes breaks taboos. The characters are generally stock figures, undifferentiated characters from the everyman Mr. Smith or Farmer Jones to the Dumb Blonde. These are short, short stories at the longest, a riddle or quick pun at the shortest.

Although the subject matter of jokes can range widely through the implausible and fantastic, the verbal forms are often quite traditional. Plots are simple and linear (no subplots, no flashbacks) with conventional developments of conflict and then a quick resolution, often in a punch line. For Aristotle, dramatic plots were logical and hinged on characters' motivations; plotlines for modern, realistic literature are usually logical, depending on linear causation. By contrast, causation in jokes is often whimsical, even bizarre, following Green World freedom, not common sense; Holt calls this, sensibly enough, "crazy logic" (p. 107).

Madelijn Strick et al. have analyzed the mental process of reading or hearing a joke: "The typical joke contains a set up that causes perceivers to make a prediction about the likely outcome. The punch line violates these expectations, and perceivers look for a cognitive rule that makes the punch line follow from the set up." Using concepts from psychology and neuroscience, these investigators further suggest that there are two mental processes at work, one affective and one rational: "...before activation of the brain's reward system (i.e., the affective response resulting from the perceived funniness of the joke), humor first activates brain areas that are associated with incongruity resolution," which they define as finding "a cognitive rule" to resolve the incongruity in the joke.[11] In the Party Time! joke, we recognize the erotic metaphor which incongruously redefines how the leather belts are to be used, although there may be variance among perceivers of this joke who find it emotionally satisfying. For Strick et al., jokes can lessen negative emotions, providing comfort and "consolatory effects," which appears to be the case for the nurses who used the Party Time! formula.

Attitude Adjustments: Varieties Of Consolation

Popular culture says that Happy Hour provides "attitude adjustment," a phrase that suggests we'll have a more cheery outlook on life after a drink or two. If our attitudes were depressed by work, family, finances, or the existential burdens of modern life in general, all these can quickly be *adjusted* for the better by alcohol, as if we were adjusting a thermostat or a lawnmower. We remain passive while the alcohol circulates through us and does its job.

Comedy is also a kind of attitude adjustment, but with less risk of intoxication or overdose, and also with more demands on our minds: we must attend to the narrative of a joke, a comic text, a movie, or a play. We make an effort to perceive the characters, the story, the images, the language, and the mood involved, and we allow our minds to play with all these elements. We make guesses about how the punch line will arrive; we enjoy how a comic narrative playfully departs from ordinary causations and descriptions. As we bring our attention and our intentions to the game of the story, our attitudes become adjusted because we affirm the notions of freedom, agency, and pleasure.

JOKERS CAN HEAL US   *High RISK*

Jokers heal us in several ways, by (1) naming (however indirectly) of things we fear, therefore (2) giving us a sense of control and (3) allowing us to deal with our emotions, and (4) inviting us to feel solidarity with others with whom we share the jokes. At their extreme, as in Party Time!, jokers may go beyond ordinary norms of speech in order to deal with difficult subjects, "outflanking" them, so to speak. Such jokers and their listeners feel solidarity within their comic community, although outsiders may find their language inappropriate or even appalling.

Jokers provide a kind of preventive medicine for their specific comic communities, allowing members to deal with worries about illness, accident, injury, loss of function, loss of looks, and death. There are also affirmations of vitality, human comradeship, imagination, and the freedoms afforded by joking. And, of course, we may feel pleasure in an exchange of jokes with jokers. Because jokers have a very wide range, it's important that the kind of joking match the expectations of the listeners. A sophisticated audience doesn't want to hear infantile prattle. A mourning person doesn't want to hear jokes about people dying. A visitor to a hospital doesn't want to hear medical students making fun of a fat patient. Jokers are sometimes high-risk comedians, but clowns are safer because we generally know what to expect.

CLOWNS CAN HEAL US

Clowns invite us into their Green World to be healed by rejoining a vibrant and healthy society. A clown in a hospital connects patients to past, presumably happy experiences. Hospital clowns are gentle and kind; they humanize and socialize the space they are in, whether a patient's room or a hallway, even an elevator car. Regrettably, the hospital world is often gray: institutional buildings, with bright fluorescent lighting—because these are deficient in red, they make everyone look gray—linoleum floors, and long hallways that look the same on every floor; the rooms, typically painted white, appear interchangeable. Such details owe to inexpensive construction, ease of maintenance, and traditions in design that lack imagination and an awareness of the personhood of patients, thus making them feel like raw material in a factory. Fortunately such norms are changing in many hospitals.

But even in the most hospitable of hospitals, a patient feels removed from home, family, friends, and other comforts of daily life, a removal that may contribute to sadness and alienation, loneliness, even fear. Clowns bring reconnection to the outside world, especially the happy world of circuses or a children's birthday party; they are instantly recognizable as figures of fun and energy, robust health, and cheerful wellness. Patients perceive them and, in varying degrees, feel positive emotions of health and happiness.

The following chart gives an idea of the wide range of jokers as opposed to the more focused roles of hospital clowns.

FIGURE 4.2: COMPARISON OF JOKERS AND HOSPITAL CLOWNS

	JOKER	HOSPITAL CLOWN
IMAGERY	Literary; wildly various	Clown garb, makeup
PRESENCE	In person, on paper, etc.	Hospital hall, room
CHARACTER(S)	Lit. types, exaggerations	Known, recognizable
COHERENCE	Imaginative leaps	Much coherence
STORY	Often a strict formula, or not	Improvisational
ENERGY	Various, even chaotic	Modulated
AUDIENCE RESPONSES	Chuckles to raucous laughter	Smiles, gentle laughter
SYMBOLIC GESTURE	A poke in the ribs, slap on the back	A gentle touch
BASIC MOOD	Various: hilarity, sarcasm, irony	Comfort

IRONY IN LIFE, IN LITERATURE

The last category, "basic mood," needs some further discussion, especially the notions of irony and comfort, two contrasting emotions that can contribute strongly to the sweet-and-sour sauce of comedy.

In the original Greek, *eiron* meant speech, but especially dissembling speech. Such activity is not news, because we routinely tell white lies, speak politely to people we don't like, and change the topic to avoid stating our true feelings. On a wider level, we all harbor ideals and goals, some of which will never be met, thus creating an ironic distance between the ideal and the actual. Still more abstractly, human life itself is pervasively ironic because all of our wishes and ideals cannot be fulfilled and, further, we are all mortals who will suffer debility and death. Various cultures deal with this fact in different ways, some celebrating the two cooperating realms, life on earth and the life beyond this one—some ignoring the discrepancy, perhaps hoping it will go away.

A thumbnail definition for ironic speech is "one thing is said but another meant"; underneath the basic meanings of the words, there is another, contrasting idea. While "irony" may sound like an abstract literary concept, ironic comments are a stuff of daily life: these come naturally to us. We routinely attack ideas, events, and people by saying the opposite of what we mean. Consider the following:

"I'm so looking forward to my next dentist appointment/mammogram/colonoscopy."

"Of course it rained: I just washed my car."

"My car made a stupid noise all the way to the garage where, of course, the noise completely disappeared."

"I told my son to be home at midnight, which, of course, he missed by two hours."

"Isn't it great that Jim Carrey/Chevy Chase/Adam Sandler is going to make another moronic movie?"

"No good deed goes unpunished."

Someone complains at length about a topic; a listener says, "Tell me how you really feel."

Or the all-purpose introductory phrase: "Don't you just love it when…."

Listeners immediately understand this verbal subterfuge, this game of saying the opposite of what we really mean, and others quickly fill in the gaps. We routinely make jokes about things that aren't going right, that don't match up with the ideal. "Just my good luck!" we ironically say about bad weather on a day we had an outdoor activity scheduled, and anyone listening understands the humor involved. Such speakers and listeners form an ad hoc comic community and share an intentional agreement that the ideal and the actual are some distance apart and that this gap is unfair.

When I taught literature, my students liked (and often actually remembered) this example of irony: *the firehouse burned down.* Here an ideal (fighting fires elsewhere, keeping a community safe) is undermined by a fire that destroys the very structure that made that ideal achievable: the absurd intrudes on social order, much as illness intrudes on a healthy person's life. No accident or illness seems to arrive at a good time; our lives typically have routines, plans, and goals. When these are abridged, there's an ironic gap. Sometimes we use humor to address the unfairness. "Just my luck to get a cold right before my performance/interview/big date!

FIGURE 4.3: IRONIC DISTANCE

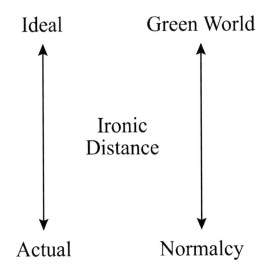

In Chapter One, we discussed the *direction* of a person wishing to join a social group: inwards for the comic movement and outwards for the tragic movement. In this chapter we're considering irony, which focuses on the *distance* between an ideal and the actual state of affairs. Irony is a tension, a distance that can be humorous, as in a routine joke that the reason there's rain is that we just washed our car, or that can be tragic and frightening, as in a sudden medical diagnosis, or in an actual burning down of a fire house, or the deaths of all the firemen from various firehouses during 9/11.

We can illustrate irony as an outward, centrifugal force and comedy as an inward, centripetal force.

These two directions provide both tension and resolution, depending on how they're used. They keep us interested in the story: we wonder how can such disparities be resolved?

FIGURE 4.4: DIRECTIONS IN IRONY AND COMFORT

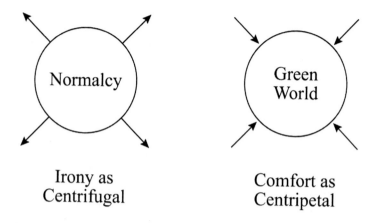

Irony as
Centrifugal

Comfort as
Centripetal

THE INTERTWINING QUALITIES OF IRONY AND COMFORT

Knock knock!

Who's there?

Influenza!

Influenza who?

I opened the window and in flew Enza!

Many will recall this knock knock joke from decades ago. It uses a child's formula that verbally domesticates influenza or, as we more commonly know it, the flu. Ordinary flu can be unpleasant enough, but other versions can be quite dangerous, killing millions of people, as in the Spanish flu pandemic of 1918-1919. In 2009-10 there was much concern about the threat of H1N1 or Swine Flu that threatened the globe. (The word "influenza" dates from medieval times, when it was assumed that illness came from the *influence* of evil stars, truly a cosmic conspiracy.) The knock knock joke creates an ironic distance away from the dangerous illness and gives us the comforts of language play and a sense of Word Magic control.

There's even a structural irony in two people telling jokes; they have agreed to leave the world of work, duty, and seriousness for the comic world where words, characters, and stories have their own imaginative reality. But in this jump to the comic world, there is also comfort because the participants share an intention: they have agreed to join in pleasurable foolishness, even a foolishness that deals with serious topics.

In ironic humor, jokers make jokes by means of a wide range of language, imagery, and subject matter. Jokers are often secure within their immediate society, but they may use ironic humor to give voice to repressed fears about subjects generally considered taboo. However crude, ironic humor is a kind of preventive medicine. Sometimes ironic jokers use many and harsh jokes which are repellent; such jokers come across as cynics who are unable to affirm anything. We tend to scapegoat them as undesirable.

The dynamics of *comfort* are somewhat different. Indeed "comfort" is surely one of the more pleasant words in our language. We think of comfort zones, comfort levels, and comfort foods; large quilts called comforters. In Handel's *Messiah*, the tenor sings, "speak ye comfortably to Jerusalem," and the refrain of a Christmas carol proclaims "tidings of comfort and joy." The Holy Spirit has been called the "Comforter." While irony plays with awkward separations and distances, comfort celebrates pleasurable togetherness. The word roots are Latin *cum* (with, together) and *fortis* (strong), suggesting that there is strength in groups of people, even people and places, even people and higher spirits. Such combinations allow us to be comfortable or even "comfy." Here we have another version of the Green World, a place where we feel contexted, happy, and fruitful. Humans love comfort because the intentions of all parties are aligned in intimacy and trust; we have a primal urge for comfort, which is a bedrock for comedy. In his movies and theme parks, Walt Disney extolled comfy togetherness, and crowds came, decade after decade. For better or worse, many Americans tend to see themselves made comfortable by a commercially Green World, a world ever more material, sensual, and pleasurable—with more money, more services, more security, more power, more health, more youth, more sex, and/or more excitement. Such a world may be as superficially green as the folding money we ordinarily use.

Our language is full of words beginning with "com," and many of these are culturally powerful: *command, commemorate, commensurate, comment, commercial, communication, community, commitment,* and many more. ("Comedy," however, is not one of them; the usual Greek origins given by dictionaries are *komos* (revel) and *aoidos* (song), meaning, roughly, a musical party.)

A fifteenth century French proverb speaks of the importance of comfort, whether or not curing is possible:

Guerir quelquefois,	To heal sometimes,
Solager souvent,	To relieve often,
Consoler toujours.	To comfort always.

We may illustrate the direction of comfort as inward, an energy directed toward the center. The periphery is a gray, threatening anarchy, where irony comprises both the impossible ideal and the anarchic. When we want comfort, we head toward a central Green World, or, more simply, *home*.

But homes can be claustrophobic and utopias can be boring, even Dante's *Paradiso*. Readers much prefer Dante's *Inferno*, where the ironic distance between sinful activity and principled punishment takes dramatic forms. Of course, armchair reading about hell and its torments can be pleasurable, an esthetic adventure undertaken in comfortable surroundings where we'd prefer to be—as opposed to being in hell itself. On the other hand, when we are too comfortable, we like some ironic variety to spark things up. The circus skillfully supplies both. Many acts provide festive and predictable events for spectators gathered together under the big top: music, cotton candy, and the lavish spectacle. But there is also potential danger in the form of elephants, tigers, and lions. When the high wire acrobat almost falls, there is a communal gasp, a communal recognition of an ironic tension between safety and danger. Clowns, as we've said, provide both comfortable and ironic spectacles, in the routine foolishness we expect but also athletic pratfalls and mock fights that never cause harm. Comedy uses comfort and irony in different proportions at different times, from the gentle nursery rhymes to sarcastic attacks, and jokers can perform at any level, taking higher risks. Hospital clowns, of course, deal in comfortable humor that likely will offend no one and also please many people, even total strangers.

Levity And Gravity: The Triumph And Failure Of Figure 4.5

"Lighten up!" we urge a melancholic person. Or we try to "make light of" our difficulties, hoping to "rise above" dilemmas at hand, which may seem grave and "weigh us down." Jokers and clowns can lift our moods from the gravity of many things, even injury and illness.

We can illustrate some of the concepts of this chapter in the following chart.

FIGURE 4.5: OVERVIEW OF COMIC FEATURES

CHARACTER/ EXAMPLE	AUDIENCE	TONE	STYLE	UNDERLYING METAPHORS	HEALING PURPOSE
Vonnie (Clown)	Hospital patients (asymmetrical)	Gentle	Improv comedy	Circus (Festive escape)	Comfort
Party Time! (Joker)	ER coworkers (symmetrical)	Harsh	Code	Erotic bondage (Sexual escape)	Ironic solidarity Cope with stress
Jokes (via email)	Social peers at leisure (symmetrical, but distant)	Varies	Written	Verbal play (Literary escape)	Pleasure Entertainment
Jokes (spoken)	Social peers at leisure (symmetrical, and present)	Varies	Oral	Verbal play (Literary performance, Social escape)	Pleasure Entertainment Social ritual

The comparatist in me is immediately pleased with this chart, all taxonomic and four-square. Some more nebulous features are not present, however, so I know it's only suggestive. Figure 4.5 is rectilinear and planar in two dimensions, like a playing card flat on the table. If we play with this model, we can consider something three-dimensional, with features above and below. Figure 4.6 shows a side view of the Overview (reduced to a single line) with three clouds, Freedom, Agency, and Joy above. We may consider these Aspirational Drives, or motivations. This is the realm of levity or lightness, and it ties directly into the various *escapes* in the Underlying Metaphors of Figure 4.5. Jokes lift us off the mundane table top, giving us pleasure in the exercise of our imaginations.

Below, we have the Solid Footing of various bedrocks; this is the realm of Gravity, rootedness, or earthiness. These include Social Solidarity, Sex, and all the features under Figure 4.5's Healing Purpose, especially Comfort, Entertainment, and Pleasure.

It would be tempting to skewer the grid with a vertical line and consider it a linear spectrum so we could place kinds of humor higher or lower, but that won't work because jokes use the higher and lower resources discontinuously, often bringing disparate ideas, images, and words together. In one sense, the higher and lower resources embrace joking and clowning, so we might think of bilocality, a concept from quantum physics that means an object can be in two places simultaneously; a pun is similar, holding two disparate meanings at once. Or we might think of curved space, which would allow the two poles of the Aspirational Drives and the Solid Footing to overlap in the Green World of love. Vonnie brings patients feelings of freedom and joy, perhaps even agency as they participate in the friendly banter of social equals. Besides these "higher" qualities, however, are also "lower" references to bowel regularity, a physician's bloody nose, and the demeaning aspects of hospital gowns and food.

FIGURE 4.6: OVERVIEW FLAT ON THE TABLE PLUS LEVITY AND GRAVITY

Levity: Aspirational Drives
Freedom, Agency, Joy

OVERVIEW → ———————————————

Gravity: Solid Footing
Social Solidarity, Sex, Comfort
Entertainment, Pleasure

Our review of the many kinds and purposes of comedy completed, Chapters Five through Nine will explore vignettes from hospitals and clinics as well as jokes, arranged according to the five qualities identified in Chapter Three: (1) taboo language, (2) imagery, (3) character and story, (4) Freudian attack, and (5) aging and death; a sixth, ritual, is pervasive because we can imagine the social contexts for these vignettes and jokes.

Chapter Five

Talking Past Taboo

When Language Mentions the Unmentionable

THE LAUNDRY CHUTE IN A PEDS WARD:

A pediatric ward in a Midwestern hospital treated sick children. Many of them made good progress and went home. Some diabetics returned now and then, but they stayed fairly stable. Indeed, one of the joys of pediatric care is seeing children who, when medically assisted, can heal and have future lives. With a patient like Ernie, however, the associations were just the opposite. He was a victim of a near-drowning, underwater for thirty minutes before he was pulled out. He survived—in the limited sense that his brain stem still fired his heart and respiration—but his higher brain was gone. As one nurse put it, "If you look into his eyes, you can see that there's nobody home." His condition was known as "persistent vegetative state," or PVS. I remember seeing a near-drowning victim in my hospital in Florida, where pediatric accidents with swimming pools, bays, rivers, and salt water are all too common. I looked into a child's beautiful blue eyes and saw, indeed, that "nobody was home."

Ernie lay in his bed day after day, week after week, month after month. For the staff working with Ernie, there was a magical hope that he'd wake up and be well but also the medical knowledge and experience that his higher brain was almost certainly completely gone and that there was no hope for him getting better, let alone having a normal childhood. The better part of a year elapsed. Cases such as these are painful and bioethically complex; many will recall the political turmoil around the Terri Schiavo case in 2005. Furthermore, in this jurisdiction there was no legal provision for removal of life support. While healthcare personnel provided professional care, they felt frustration and even anger at the hopelessness of the case. Nevertheless, they fulfilled their duties and kept their feelings to themselves.

One day a nurse was dragging a sack of laundry across the floor, heading for the laundry chute. Suddenly he burst into a ventriloquist routine, as if the laundry were speaking.

In a falsetto approximating a child's voice, he cried out, "No, no, don't put me in the laundry chute!"

He then spoke in his own voice, "It's OK, Ernie."

"No, no, don't put me there!"

"But Ernie, you know this is best for you."

"But no, no, no, don't do this!"

"Yes, Ernie, I'm sorry, but we're going to do away with you now!"

"No, no no!"

"Yes, yes, yes!"

Startled nurses and doctors looked and listened. Some burst into laughter. Some chuckled and shook their heads. Others looked away.

The nurse had broken the professional taboo of not mentioning the futility of Ernie's state and, worse, the social and legal taboo against killing patients. And yet this ferocious, ironic humor gave voice to long unspoken feelings, broke the tension of repressing them, and—to some extent—helped the staff to continue with daily care of Ernie. The nurse's role as joker worked (at least for some of his colleagues) because of the shared values of their particular subculture and the creativity of his joke that allowed for a semblance of a comic community. (Whether the nurse understood himself to be a joker or was driven by the turmoil in his unconscious, we'll never know.)

When, at last, Ernie's heart failed on its own, there was both sadness and relief.

JOKES AND LANGUAGE PLAY

Many jokes play with language, showing it to be ambiguous and suggestive in odd ways that sometimes break taboos. Here are two examples.

Doctor to elderly woman: "How long have you been bedridden?"

Woman: "Gosh, not for about 20 years, when my husband was still alive."

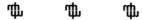

"Hello! You have reached the Incontinence Hot Line! Can you hold?"

Humans can speak to each other in many wonderful ways—and some not so wonderful. We flirt, we insult, we cajole, we give orders. We can also make light of things, tell jokes, offer obnoxious puns, and otherwise participate in a wide range of humor. Words are the artistic medium of jokes, much as paint or steel are media for painters and sculptors, and language has a very wide range of meanings and moods, from the most exalted and lyrical words to earthy and rude ones. Language that breaks taboo includes so-called dirty words but also words that have double meanings. Sometimes a dirty word is an expletive used in anger. Sometimes it is a marker of friendship for a particular group. I recall making repairs with a relative who swore freely as we worked, but he never used such language with his family. Similarly, a nurse swore freely at her computer, but she always spoke formally with patients.

Language is not as specific or efficient as we like to think; puns are a good example of failure in language. In *On Puns: The Foundation of Letters*, Jonathan Culler calls puns "lively instances of lateral thinking, exploiting the fact that language has ideas of its own" (p. 15).[1] If we can consider language to be personified in this way, language enjoys participating in jokes because jokes draw attention to the sounds of words, the ambiguities of words, even downright failures of language to be exact. (The morning newspaper reports that the comedian Gallagher wants an added dial for his TV so he can increase intelligence of programming; he declares that he's tried the dial for "Brightness," and it didn't work.) Some people don't like puns because of this treachery, and many people will offer a groan as the conventional response. But some people enjoy fooling with the slipperiness of words, even words that speak to basic human conditions such as health and illness, physical appearance and ability, sexual matters, and death.

In the Incontinence Hot Line joke above, we can see that three important things happen in the activity of the joke. First, we've moved the topic of urinary incontinence from the (usually) unspoken realm of taboo to the spoken realm of recognition; the joke brings something hidden into specific, named consideration. Second, the joke has a frame of familiarity because it uses two literary forms, a parody of the all-too-familiar outgoing telephone message and the literary form of a pun ("hold"), a single word in which two meanings collide; perhaps we groan at this pun because we know one when we see one, and we realize immediately that a joke is being made. Third, the joke treats the subject with a mood of joking, of humor, of satire. Jokes of all kinds have the power to change mood, to shift our emotions, to cast a different perspective on some topic. Incontinence is ordinarily a distressing topic, one that suggests frustration, shame, and physical and emotional discomfort. After all, one of our first successes as young children is mastering toilet training; as adults, we take pride (if only on a subconscious level) in being able to manage our bladder and bowels. To go backwards in this skill is demeaning to us, a sense that we're "over the hill" and headed downwards, perhaps even toward death. By poking fun at incontinence, however, we can claim—if just for the moment—control over the topic and our emotional response to it.

In this chapter, we will look at some aspects of language that are central to medical jokes: (1) taboo, (2) puns and other word play, and—of course!—(3) medical terms, although these categories will inevitably overlap each other.

Fred &
WILMA IN bed

NICE TALK AND NOT-NICE TALK: THE SHIFTING BORDERS OF TABOO

Taboos can change within a culture over time. Going back a generation or two, the term "unmentionables" meant underwear, items that could not be talked about, clothing that was physically near—even touched!—organs of sex and elimination. Today, the taboos have shifted so that underclothing is no longer taboo; indeed some fashions in clothing routinely show bra straps and the tops of boxer shorts. On the other hand, jokes using urine or feces still have power because of taboos; here's a joke that includes an element of revolt against a medical gatekeeper:

Waiting Room Propriety

A man walks up to the receptionist's desk in a crowded waiting room.

She says, "Yes, sir, what can we do for you today?"

He says, first looking around nervously at other patients, "Well, it's about my dick," he finishes in a whisper.

"Your what?" she says, "Come, speak up; I can hardly hear you!"

"My dick," he says a bit louder. Everyone stares at him.

"I'm sorry, sir, but we can't have that kind of language in this office. Please go out the door, come back in, and try again."

The man leaves.

He returns.

He approaches the desk.

"Yes?" she says.

"It's about my ear," he says.

"That's much better," she says, nodding with approval.

"And just what's wrong with your ear?"

"I can't piss out of it!"

In this joke, the male and female character fight using language as weaponry. First, of course, is the woman's proclamation of taboo, her challenge as a gatekeeper, with the reinforcing factor of an audience in the waiting room: by making the man speak up, she shames him before strangers. She is a classic figure, a self-appointed enforcer of norms—a Mrs. Grundy, a castrating bitch, a Nurse Ratched from Ken Kesey's novel *One Flew over the Cuckoo's Nest* (1962). She reminds us of teachers (many of them women) who corrected or punished us in our youths—not to mention the disciplining roles of our mothers. She is a satiric extreme, of course, especially in her correction of the relatively mild word "dick," and certainly in the absurd use of the grade-school ritual she puts the man through (to leave and return). Yet the shame of patients caused by gatekeepers, insurance forms, referrals, personal questions asked in public, and the like is well known. I can recall being asked for the date of a diagnosis for my cancer in a semi-public space every time I visited a clinic. Sometimes people speak loudly to a patient, as if the patient is deaf (or stupid) as well as sick. Sometimes there's a low- or middle-level manager with little internal power who exercises limited authority upon clients and customers in abusive ways. Sometimes an office worker is bound by policy and can act no other way.

Our unnamed receptionist reproves the man as if he were a naughty little boy, infantalizing him, on a day when, we may assume, he already feels terrible. He has a sexual ailment for which she has no sympathy, and, worse, she is eager to have it described for all present. When he outfoxes her (at least for the moment; do we consider that he improved his standing within that office?), we feel a vengeance has been rightly meted out on behalf of all of us who have been unjustly pushed around, especially by officious and self-aggrandizing women (or men). In my experience, however, women hearing this joke seem to laugh just as hard as men, identifying with the patient not so much because he is a man but because he is a victim of bureaucratic nonsense.

The punch line provides the man's revenge, initially through his subterfuge of the safe word "ear" and then the hammer-blow of the word "piss," several levels worse than "dick." Through the symbolic power of taboo speech, he has publicly pissed on her, judging her, her waiting room, her Miss Priss ethos, and her power games.

It's been said that women are the guardians of nice manners, nice speech, and polite society in general, while men are the oafs, the grunts, the crudes. It has also been suggested that women—typically of smaller stature than men—use their tongue as their weapon. (Brain function studies have shown women to have larger and more active language areas; they tend to excel on standardized exams in verbal tests, while men often do better in mathematics.) Men tend to favor the more crude, gross, and bizarre jokes, while women especially like jokes that hinge on word play and character interaction. If such a generalization may be entertained (and we know there are many exceptions), these suggest two interactive and often reinforcing poles of humor: language play (this chapter) and outlandish images (the next chapter).

EUPHEMISMS

A euphemism is a word or a phrase that refers to an unpleasant or taboo subject indirectly, so as to avoid emotional meanings of more direct words. (The Greek roots are *eu* meaning "good," "well," or "pleasing" and *pheme* meaning "speech.") In the ER, the phrase "unrestrained passengers" meant people not wearing seatbelts—and certainly not "people who are emotionally free." This phrase often came over the radio when car wreck victims were coming to us. The phrase is euphemistic, because it masks the violent images of injury, especially for children, who can be tossed around a car or a van with serious—and largely avoidable—injuries. ER personnel don't like to hear the phrase, because they know what danger lies hidden underneath the many neutral-sounding syllables.

Often a euphemism is an attempt to get around a taboo, for example against "dirty" words. The Waiting Room Propriety joke illustrates the tension between formal levels of language (female-dominated in this example) and less formal, or slang level. Taboo often provides a dividing line to suppress references in "bad" language to body parts, bodily excretions, and other nastinesses—including death. A solution is often euphemism, or a "nice way" of verbalizing any unsavory subject. The following joke presents female, animal characters (theriomorphs) with human qualities:

Two cows are standing next to each other in a field.

Daisy says to Dolly, "Well, what's new?"

Dolly says, "Oh not, much. How about you?"

"Well, did you see the vet's van here this morning?"

"Come to think of it, I did."

"Yes, well, it was here. And guess what? I was artificially inseminated."

"No way! I don't believe you," says Dolly.

"But it's true," Daisy exclaims. "Very easy. In fact, no bull!"

And the cows share a quiet laugh.

Here the pun "no bull" conflates "I'm telling the truth" (literally, no bullshit in euphemized form) with the sly suggestion that male participants in sex are annoying or troublesome.

A more elaborate joke from the veterinarian world involves husband-wife acrimony:

A man buys a large and very expense Rottweiler and takes it home to show off to his wife.

"Look at this fine beast," he extols.

She looks him over and complains, "But it's cross-eyed!"

"It's not."

"It is."

They argue for a time, but finally the man looks more closely and is horrified to see that his wife is correct. He phones the seller and complains, but to no avail.

He takes the dog to the vet. In the exam room the man and the vet heave the dog up onto the stainless steel table.

The vet looks him over and says, "Well, yes, this dog is indeed cross-eyed. You're going to have to put him down."

"What!" cries the man, "Just because he's cross-eyed?"

"No, because he weighs 105 pounds. I'm afraid I'll hurt my back!"

In this joke, the euphemistic idiom for killing (or "putting to sleep" or "euthanizing") an animal is disassembled to its literal parts.

Ironically enough, euphemisms can actually draw attention to the word being avoided: The autonomic system of the brain controls the four "F"s: Feeding, Fighting, Fleeing, and Reproduction.

Women, of course, aren't the only euphemizers, as in the following joke.

A lazy man finally visits his doctor; his wife has been nagging him for months to have a physical because of his general lassitude.

The doctor checks him from stem to stern and finds nothing wrong.

He says, "Well Mr. Smith, it seems that there's nothing physical holding you back. I guess I'd just have to say you're lazy."

"I know, I know," says Mr. Smith. "But give me the medical term so I can tell my wife."

In this case, the common word "lazy" is taboo for Mr. Smith, who wants the camouflage of medical obfuscation. Perhaps the appropriate humour word "phlegmatic" would have satisfied him.

RELIGION AND TABOO

While many contemporary American jokes use taboos against the "lower" bodily parts and functions, the original sense of taboo to hide higher religious matters has not died out entirely. "Thou shalt not take the name of the LORD in vain" is one of the Ten Commandments, meaning we shouldn't say "God" (or Yahweh or Jehovah) for a trifling purpose, such as voicing pain after stubbing one or more of our toes.

Indeed, one of the functions of humor is to reunite the two extremes that run from the basement of the excremental and the sexual to the highest heavens of the formal, abstract, and spiritual, as we were saying with the Clouds of Aspiration and the Solid Footings in Figure 4.6. This is not a new idea, but one for which we need reminders, especially in this culture, strongly influenced by Puritanism. There is a long tradition in the joke world of opposing priests, nuns, ministers, etc. to the realms of the flesh, but sometimes allowing the two to overlap. In the following joke the Pope is characterized as having a mind as slangy and racy as "the rest of us." Or, in the popular phrase, "Even the Pope puts on his pants every morning." Or, as attributed to Montaigne, "No matter how high up [in society] you sit, you always sit on your ass." In the world of comedy, we are all fundamentally the same. In different times there are different taboos: Chaucer used the word "cunt" (spelled "queynte") in *The Canterbury Tales*, often with a pun on the word we spell today as "quaint."

The Pope Near Death

Although not particularly old—at least by Papal standards—the Pope is dying. Vatican physicians find no overt cause. Celebrated doctors from across Italy are, likewise, stumped. [Versions variously pursue different medical authorities, satirizing different specialties, nationalities, bioethical persuasions, etc., depending on how shaggily and/or tediously the joke is constructed.]

The cardinals are desperate; finally they call on a woman from the mountains known for her psychic abilities.

She arrives, looks at the Pope, and goes into a trance.

Upon emerging, she utters an unintelligible oracle and smiles, as if all were solved.

The cardinals ask her to explain in plain language.

"I said, it's a clear case of DSI."

"What?" everyone asks.

"Deadly Seminal Impaction."

She tries to leave.

"But wait! What is the treatment?"

"There is none, except of course, the obvious sexual relations which will put him back in the pink."

"But this is the Pope!"

"I know." She raises an admonitory finger, widens her eyes, and intones, "You must choose whether he'll serve the Church better on earth or in Heaven!"

"Of course. I suppose manual stimulation is out of the question."

"Clearly inadequate. Certain deeper areas of the brain must be stimulated."

The cardinals debate all this in protracted fashion then lay all the options before his Holiness.

He too has extreme reservations and will not hear of the proposed course of treatment. But, when exhorted to consider his role in the church and so forth, he ponders, prays, ruminates, and finally speaks.

"I can consent to such radical treatment only if three conditions are met."

"Yes?"

"Number One: she must be blind, so that she cannot see who her partner might be in this radical therapeutic intervention."

"It shall be done."

"Number Two: she must be deaf, to guard against the slightest chance that His Eminence might inadvertently utter even the briefest of inchoate sounds such as might betray not only his identity but also his pleasure."

"It shall be done. And...number three, your Holiness?"

"Number three, ah yes. Big tits!"

Here again, one of the holiest of men is characterized as needing not only sexual release but sexual enjoyment—topics often taboo in polite society. The Pope, a symbol of things holy and distant, is drawn (partially against his Holy will) back "down" into the wider circle of earthy humanity.

This joke parallels other jokes in which a clownish figure names three conditions, the third being non-parallel and climactically ridiculous. In this joke, the third demand emphasizes the Pope's hidden (taboo) interest in women and sexuality. By suddenly revealing his hidden earthy, animal side, he balances—at least to the generic popular mind—his phlegmatic humour with his repressed sanguine humour. The Pope here represents repressions about sexuality in general, and we may find relief in the joke's affirmation that everyone normally has sexual urges and instincts, which, finally, should be accepted and even celebrated. It's important also that all the cardinals (men) and doctors (presumably men) have failed to help the Pope; by contrast, a wise old woman, a crone, knows the physical-psychological-spiritual truth of the matter and names the healing course of action.

In a wider sense, humor often has values that are judgmental and demanding. In this joke, we find a problematic, universal declaration that all people (namely men) must have sex (and heterosexual sex, not homosexual, not masturbatory sex). While comedy often shows an urge within society to reproduce itself, there can be a demanding, even fascist side to comedy, a single right way to act. Humor can carry not only conventional values, but even monolithic ones.

Another joke with a clerical character illustrates taboo in another way; the joke must date back some years, since it concerns not one doctor but two doctors actually making house calls:

A Doctor Starting Out

Just out of training, a young doctor moves to a small community to replace the doctor who is retiring. As part of the transfer of the practice, the young doc-

Getting to Know
for us a key to I___

tor is to observe the doc's office visits for two weeks and to accompany him on the house calls.

At one household the pair arrives and the older doctor interviews the woman, who is in bed. She complains of bowel distress, diarrhea, flatulence, and so on.

The older doctor says, "Well, you're basically in good health. It's just that you've been overdoing fresh fruit, and I think you need to cut back on that."

She thanks him warmly, and the two docs depart.

As they travel to the next household, the young doctor says, "Say, doctor, I certainly admire the speed of your diagnosis, but you didn't even examine her, let alone take a full history. Shouldn't your differential diagnosis be a bit longer before coming to a treating diagnosis?"

The older doc smiles to himself and thinks about the whipper-snappers of today and their inadequate training. Nonetheless, he patiently explains.

"Well, I know you are all versed today in evidence-based medicine, randomized control studies, case-matched comparisons, and so on, but there's really no getting around local lore, knowing your patients, and tricks of the trade."

"Gosh...really? So how did that work with that patient?"

"Well, at her house, while I was sitting down, I dropped my stethoscope. When I reached down to pick it up, I looked under the bed and noticed a large pile of fruits peelings, cores, and seeds. Clearly that was the behavioral background I needed. The diagnosis was not only easy but also right as rain."

"Saved you a lot of time too!" the young doc enthused.

At the next house, the older doc suggests that the young doc take the lead and put his recent learning to work. Accordingly, he asked the sick woman how she felt.

"I just don't seem to have the same energy," she said. "I get tired in the evenings. My husband says I'm not much of a wife to him anymore because I'm so run down."

"Well, then, I'd suggest you cut back on church work. I'm confident your energy will rebound."

She thanked him warmly, and the doctors departed.

As they drove on to next stop, the older doc said, "I'm sure your diagnosis was correct. And it certainly was quick. Just fill me in on how you reached it."

"Certainly. I followed your instructions carefully. I dropped the stethoscope. When I stooped down to pick it up, I noticed the preacher under the bed."

This is a thoroughly silly story in its abandonment of standard medical process, but it well illustrates the conventional taboo about a religious figure and sex. It also emphasizes a doctor's participation in the private affairs of his or her patients, here presented in the imagery of a bedroom farce. In both visits, the doctors not only "see" the patient in the idiomatic sense ("We're seeing a lot of colds this season") but also in the literal sense of seeing fruit detritus and a preacher, visual symbols of excess in the lives of the two patients. Indeed, a doctor sees a lot of our bodies and our lives. On the one hand, we're thankful for this, since such seeing leads to diagnosis and treatment. On the other hand, we may resent it, because our modesty and privacy are abridged and because we are seen in all our weakness and vulnerability.

The social function of taboo is to acknowledge the power (for Polynesians, the "mana") of the taboo material, for example the importance of sex or God Almighty. Jokes crossing the taboo line can gain considerable energy from the taboo, although the nature of the audience will be crucial to the outcome. At an extreme, there are comedians who are so foul-mouthed that some listeners will not enjoy any of their humor; on the other hand, grade-schoolers may ritually laugh at a joke that has a dirty word in the punch line, even if the rest of the joke is not funny or even intelligible.

We can also think of taboos that comics have imposed upon themselves. When AIDS came upon the American scene in the 1980s, there were some AIDS jokes, often of the sick or macabre sort. (The AIDS diet at the hospital was said to be flounder and pancakes, the two things you could slide under the door without seeing the patient.) As professional comedians recognized that many people in show business were ill with AIDS, they agreed to make the topic thoroughly taboo. Ordinary jokers have also avoided AIDS jokes as well. For most people now, it seems that AIDS is completely taboo as a subject for humor. (Furthermore—and regrettably—for some people, AIDS is also taboo even for political and educational action.)

While there are plenty of jokes about menopause and other aspects of aging (see Chapter Nine), in my collecting I have found almost none about menstruation and ejaculation. These two bodily functions seem to remain largely taboo, although there are plenty of jokes about hot flashes and impotence.

GROANS FOR THE "LOWEST FORM OF HUMOR," PUNS, AND OTHER PLAYS ON WORDS

Another resource for humor is the pun, a word that brings two senses of meaning together in an unlikely collision. (In some jokes, I'll give the alternative meaning in brackets; for others, I'll underline the pun in a rough approximation of how a speaker might give emphasis through changes in vocal pitch, volume, or duration in delivering the joke. A spoken version would be, of course, better nuanced.)

Did you hear about the optician who fell into his lens-grinding machine and made a *spectacle* of himself?

This one is from our British correspondents:

Patient, "Doctor, doctor, you must help me. At night, I have the terrible urge to run downstairs and stick my penis into the biscuit tin. Can you help me?"

Doctor, "Certainly. I recognize the problem right away: you're fucking crackers [quite crazy]."

🜊   🜊   🜊

"I saw a dreadful accident just outside of town today. A huge truck smashed into the corner of a car, right along the driver's side, shearing off bits of the engine, chassis, fire wall, dashboard—everything, slick as a whistle. Even the driver was cut exactly in two. He got taken to the hospital where the docs did all sorts of miraculous things, so he's doing fine now: indeed, he's *all right*."

🜊   🜊   🜊

A teenager walks into a pharmacy and nervously says, "Um, I need some, er, protection."

The kind pharmacist says, "You mean some rubbers, I take it. They're right over here. What size?"

"Oh, I guess about average, I guess."

"No problem. That'll be $5.00 plus the tax."

"Tacks? I thought rubbers stayed on by themselves!"

🜊   🜊   🜊

What's the difference between a genealogist and gynecologist? One looks up the family tree, and the other looks up the family bush.

Sometimes the humor resides in reversed words (reminiscent of the Spoonerisms that reverse initial sounds):

What's the difference between a hematologist and a urologist? A hematologist pricks your finger....

And:

A doctor is writing in a chart at the nursing station when a man screams and runs out of his hospital room. A nurse chases him with a pan of very hot water and a determined look on her face. The doctor puts down his pen and yells, "Nurse, I very clearly stated that you should prick his boil!"

We like to think that language—the words we daily use for many good purposes—makes a lot of sense, that it is orderly, that the words we use refer neatly to reality, and even that we can control reality through the language of Word Magic. But comics, writers, and scalawags of every stripe like to point out the flaws, the oddities, the vagaries of language, especially words that have not one but two or more meanings.

Comics will tell you right away that language is slippery, goofy, and fun to play with. When a spoken word can mean two different things simultaneously, the punster feels delight, and the audience groans or perhaps chuckles. Why do we call puns the lowest form of humor? Perhaps because they are short—brief explosions of foolishness—but perhaps even more, because they signal that our language is basically and irrevocably flawed in its pursuit of utility and clarity. Indeed, puns suggest a deep-rooted arbitrary nature of our language. What are we to make of a word like "number" which can mean either "more numb" or an arithmetic symbol?   Or consider: an invalid in bed who has an invalid driver's license. Or this formulation: the nurse wound the gauze around the patient's wound. These aren't jokes—yet, anyway—but they illustrate inherent oddities in our wordstock that jokesters are all too glad to raise to our attention and even to celebrate.

In the following pages, we'll look at variations on puns: medical language, coined words, dyslexic scramblings, extending punning, and ambiguous words.

Puns Based On Medical Language

Predictably, there are a good many puns using medical language, especially technical terms that ordinary folks may have trouble perceiving or saying, words that often have Latin or Greek roots, words that are often of many syllables. Medical language is a source of humor for Mark Leyner and Billy Goldberg, M.D., in their *Let's Play Doctor: The Instant Guide to Walking, Talking, and Probing Like a Real M.D.*[2]

And from the oral tradition:

How do you circumcise a whale? Send down foreskin divers [four skindivers].

Sometimes the words of a joke are ordinary, but have double meanings nonetheless:

A man goes to visit his doctor.

"I feel terrible, doc; I don't know what's come over me. I can be going along just normal and suddenly I think I'm a teepee."

"That's certainly unusual. Any other symptoms?"

"Well, sometimes I think I'm a wig-wam."

"Ah, so we're making progress here," the doctor says. "I don't think you should worry too much about this; every now and then we run across a person who is two tents [too tense]."

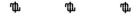

In the next joke, there's the conventional setting of a bar, with, however, some unusual characters:

Two tigers walk into a bar, take their seats, and order drinks. One tiger notices a woman at the other end and comments to his companion how attractive she is.

The other, older, and more experienced tiger says, "Oh no, you don't want to get mixed up with her type!"

Nonetheless, after another drink the younger tiger sends her a drink and the two exchange flirtatious glances.

After one more round, the younger tiger gets up and goes over and sits by her. He finds her irresistible, pounces on her, and consumes her messily but entirely. He returns to his original bar stool and downs yet another drink.

Soon he puts his large paw to his stomach and says to his friend, "I don't feel so good."

Of course not," says his friend, "and it serves you right: that was a bar bitch you ate [barbiturate]."

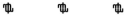

"Doctor, doctor, you must help me: I've just swallowed a pillow!"
"Good Lord, how do you feel?"
"A little *down* in the mouth."

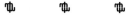

Husband's note on the kitchen table: Someone called from the Guyna College. Said the Pabst Beer [Pap smear] was normal.

🕮   🕮   🕮

A man rushed into the doctor's office and burst out, "Doctor, doctor! You must help me. I'm shrinking!"

And the doctor said, "Now calm down…you're just going to have to be a little patient."

A doctor's directions can be misunderstood even when ordinary language is used.

A woman goes to her doctor for advice about losing weight. He suggests that she follow a certain diet for two days, then skip a day, then diet, and so on. When she returns in a week, she has lost 25 pounds.

"Good heavens," says the doctor, "this result is well beyond what I envisioned."

"Me too, and I'm so happy about the weight, but my feet and knees really hurt," she says. "In fact, the first few days of skipping just about killed me."

℞   ℞   ℞

Sign on a medical school building: Staph only.

℞   ℞   ℞

The problem with the gene pool is that there is no lifeguard.

Here is a joke that has been making the rounds for a dozen years in many versions:

A man arrives at the veterinary office carrying a very limp dog. He lays the dog on the table, and the doctor puts a stethoscope on the dog's chest, in first one position than another.

"I can't seem to get a pulse here...or here...or here. I'm sorry, sir, but I must tell you that your dog has passed away."

"Oh, no!" the man cries, "That can't possibly be. I demand another opinion and right away!"

"If you insist, sir." The vet leaves the room and returns with a large black dog wearing a white coat. The dog walks up and down the table sniffing the dead dog carefully and thoroughly. Finally he lowers his own tail, sadly shakes his head, and says, "Arf" in a mournful tone.

The vet takes the Labrador out and brings back a calico cat in a custom-fit white coat. The cat similarly walks up and down the table, sniffing delicately. As before, the cat indicates, through gesture and a pitiful "Meow" that the dog has indeed expired.

"That'll be $600," says the vet.

"What?" says the man. "That's outrageous!"

"Well, if you had taken my word, it would have been $50, but with the Lab work and the CAT scan, it really adds up."

These puns are simple, even obvious, but the punch line may appeal to any patients who have paid a lot for lab services or imaging, typically billed separately from the hospital and the physician. The large additional fees also suggest that the vet has taken monetary vengeance on the man who would not believe the initial assessment. Many other jokes have hinged on the supposed greed of doctors and abuse of power, as we shall see in Chapter Eight. On the other hand, we may assume that the man with the dead dog, for example, is simultaneously angry and sad, clearly not ready to accept the obvious fact that his beloved pet has died. Because the vet did not (or could not) deal with the man's emotions, the vet and the man got into a conflict over money.

Other puns play more specifically with taboo.

A doctor is walking down the street when he sees Norm, one of the patients.

"Hey, Norm! You're looking great...so happy!"

"Yeah, doc. I feel terrific. I've found the girl of my dreams and we're engaged."

"That's wonderful! Who is the young lady?"

"Lydia Forsythe."

"Forsythe, Lydia...Lydia...Oh yes, she's one of my patients also."

A cloud passes over the doctor's face. "But my God, she has acute angina!"

Embarrassed, Norm mutters, "Well, she has a nice smile too."

Not knowing the medical terminology for chest pain, Norm does the best he can, thinking of "a cute vagina" and feeling awkward that his doctor has such intimate—and appreciative—physical knowledge of his fiancée. This joke (and many others) play on the taboo against male doctors' sexual feelings about their women patients and their presumed eagerness to be involved with them.

Indeed there are numerous jokes referring to our fears that doctors and nurses profit unethically from their positions to exploit patients sexually, as in the one-liner: Did you hear about the nurse who could make the patient without disturbing the bed? Here a traditional phrase is swapped around and the nurse is made a sexual aggressor.

Sometimes ordinary language is energized by a medical context:

A young doctor just out of medical school announced to his wife that he planned to specialize in gynecology. When she asked him why, he replied, "I've just heard there's lots of openings."

In the following joke, it's medical personnel not understanding language, and, once again, there's a religion-earth polarity:

A man is lying in bed in a Catholic hospital with an oxygen mask over his mouth. A young nurse arrives to sponge his cheeks and brow.

"Nurse," he mumbles from behind his mask, "are my testicles black?"

Horrified, the nurse stutters, "I h-have no idea. I'm here to sponge your face in order to lower your temperature."

"But this is important," he continues. "I must know: are my testicles black?"

"I don't know, sir," she says more loudly. The ward sister passing by hears her exasperated tone and looks into the room.

"Just what is going on here, nurse?" she demands.

"Um," the young nurse begins, but is interrupted by Mr. Smith, who plaintively asks once again, "Are my testicles black?"

A nurse of considerable experience and forthrightness, the ward sister whips off the sheets, rips open the man's pajamas, lifts his penis, and makes her observation.

"No, my good man, the color is normal."

Mr. Smith, using his last bit of energy, pulls off his oxygen mask and enunciates clearly, "Please, I just want to know are my test results back?"

And here's a monetary pun that has been worked two different ways:

A woman brings her son into the Emergency Room.

"Doctor, doctor, you must help me. Timmy has just swallowed a quarter!"

"Oh dear, this could be serious, but perhaps nature will take its course and the coin will just pass on through little Timmy."

She stays for a long time, worrying and fretting.

After a while, the doctor sends her home, telling her to get some rest but to call at any time for an update.

She drives home, runs to the phone, and dials the number for the ER.

"Doctor, how's little Timmy?" she cries out.

Comes the reply: "No change yet!"

"No change" puns on coinage, of course, and also a traditional medical phrase that is often disturbing for family members who are hoping for a change for the better for their loved one.

Another variation:

A woman has been passing pennies when she urinates. She explains this dilemma to her physician, who ponders the matter and suggests that she eat less copper.

A week later, she's back, complaining that nickels are now coming through.

The doctor is totally puzzled, but he suggests that they wait a week to see if the problem will resolve itself.

Next week, it's dimes.

The following week, it's quarters.

Totally stumped and, now alarmed, the doctor calls the Mayo Clinic.

"My God, you've got to help me, because it'll be 50 cent pieces next, then silver dollars!"

"Now, now," the specialist soothes, "we've seen this before. Don't concern yourself unnecessarily: she's just going through the change."

Menopause is sometimes a taboo concept—although less so in the past decade, especially with the Baby Boomers coming into middle age; now there is more frank discussion about hot flashes and the like. By making a joke about menopause, we can acknowledge that it does happen and that we can have a lighter attitude about it.

And now, appropriately enough:

Coined Words

Coined words are made up, newly minted, so to speak.
is more specifically a portmanteau word, a word that has reco
this one appeared in the Washington Post (which in itself show
have been changing over the last 25 years): an "ignoranus" is a
stupid and an asshole.

Proprietary names for drugs are usually carefully constructe
pleasant or powerful action; these are often good examples of co
example "Viagra," which suggests both "Niagara" (what a flow!), "
and "agriculture" (as in plowing). Jokers have enjoyed creating pai
pharmaceutical coinages; the following examples combine several satiri

BUYAGRA: Injectable stimulant taken prior to shopping. Increa
and duration of spending spree.

DAMNITOL: Take two and the rest of the world can go to hell
eight hours.

PEPTOBIMBO: Liquid silicone for single women. Two full cups swa
before an evening out increases breast size, improves flirting, and decreases intelligence.

DUMMEROL: When taken with Peptobimbo, can cause dangerously low I.Q. and intense enjoyment of country western music.

FUKKITOL: Powerful enema that induces disasssociation from reality for several days; recommended for all stressful situations. Contraindicated for patients already on Dammitol.

EMPTYNESTROGEN: Suppository that eliminates melancholy and loneliness by reminding you of how awful your children were as teenagers and how you couldn't wait till they moved out!

ST. MOMMA'S WORT: Plant extract that treats mom's depression by rendering preschoolers unconscious for up to two days.

FLIPITOR: Increases life expectancy of commuters by controlling road rage and the urge to flip off other drivers.

MENICILLIN: Potent anti-boy-otic for older women. Increases resistance to such lethal lines as, 'You make me want to be a better person.'

ANTI-TALKSIDENT: A spray carried in a purse or wallet to be used on anyone too eager to share their life stories with total strangers in elevators.

NAGAMENT: When administered to a boyfriend or husband, provides the same irritation level as nagging him, without opening your mouth.

JACKASSPIRIN: Relieves headache caused by a man who can't remember your birthday, anniversary, phone number, or to lift the toilet seat.

DYSLEXIA JOKES

The medical condition of dyslexia has inspired some humor, not because the illness itself is comical, but because it is an excuse to transpose letters for new meanings and show, once again, the arbitrariness of our language.

Did you hear about the dyslexic who sold his soul to Santa [Satan]?

☩   ☩   ☩

Did you hear about the dyslexic who walked into a bra?

☩   ☩   ☩

What does a dyslexic agnostic do? He stays up all night wondering if there really is a dog.

☩   ☩   ☩

What does DNA stand for? The National Dyslexia Association.

☩   ☩   ☩

What does DMA stand for? Mothers Against Dyslexia.

☩   ☩   ☩

What is the dyslexic motto? Dyslexics of the world untie!

Besides the language play involved, these jokes acknowledge that dyslexia exists and suggest that a comic perception of it is possible. On the negative side, however, dyslexics are satirized in these jokes as inept with language and scapegoated as abnormal.

Extended Puns

A shaggy dog version of a joke with puns will build a complex (and typically unlikely) narrative that ends in a series of puns that are a parody of a traditional phrase, as in "the Guru who refused Novacain at the dentist because he wanted to transcend dental medication." (For the presumed origin of shaggy dog jokes, consult this endnote.[3])

These extended jokes, with their long setups, are usually real groaners, as in the following:

A man goes to his dentist because his plate is dissolving and some of his false teeth are falling off.

Says the dentist, "I've never seen anything like this; indeed, this may be unprecedented in the dental literature. What on earth, may I ask, have you been ingesting?"

"Well, I guess I must tell you: each year, starting at Thanksgiving, I eat only dishes that have been made with Hollandaise sauce."

"Very unusual, but I think I can understand how those foodstuffs are dissolving the materials of standard dentistry. By taking a different approach, we can accommodate the dilemma associated with your lifestyle."

The man comes back next week and finds a very shiny prosthesis ready for fitting.

"Good Heavens," he says, "how come it's so shiny?"

The good dentist replies, "Simple. There's no plate like chrome for the Hollandaise."

And as for a physician's diagnosis:

Ralph and Minerva were making passionate love in a mini van, when she yelled out, "Oh, whip me! Whip me! Whip me now!"

Ralph wondered how he might do this, given that he had neither a whip nor any prospects for obtaining one. An inspiration seized him, however, and he rolled down the window and reached for the antenna. With a grunt, he snapped it off and proceeded to fulfill Minerva's request.

A few days later, Minerva sees that the cuts inflicted by the whipping are starting to fester and she presents herself to the doctor. The doctor looks her over and asks, "Did these marks occur during sex play?"

She doesn't want to answer.

He probes, "That information could be helpful to me in reaching a diagnosis and treatment."

"OK, in that case. Yes," she says and explains the situation fully.

"Just as I thought. I've only seen this in textbooks, so you are my first documentable case of van aerial disease."

Puns about the Human Body

We'll discuss physical aspects of the body in Chapter Six, but for now we can look at jokes with puns about male and female forms.

Ladies first.

Mr. Ford Speaks With God

When Henry Ford went to heaven, Saint Peter greeted him with admiration. "Mr. Ford, your numerous inventions are well known, even up here. I am authorized to grant you an interview with God Himself."

"Most kind of you," Ford replied. "And as a matter of fact, there's a design question I'd like to ask Him about."

"Well, as you know God has designed quite a number of things," said Peter with a grin. "I'm sure He'd be glad to answer your question."

"Actually, I have a complaint."

"My, my. That should be interesting."

Ford approaches the throne. After pleasantries, Ford asks, "When you designed human females, whatever were you thinking?"

"My son, I was thinking of a large number of things, including the generative activities of Adam and Eve which would lead to the human race. Why do you ask, Mr. Ford?"

"Well, frankly, I believe there are number of design flaws which should warrant reconfiguration."

"Do you now. Such as?"

"I have a little list here. First, maintenance is extremely high. Second, the rear end wobbles too much. Third, she chatters too much. Fourth, she's out of commission three or four days of the month. Fifth, the headlights are too small. Sixth, one of the intakes is placed too close to the exhaust. Seventh, she constantly needs refinishing. And there are others we could also discuss."

"Hmmm," says God. "Maybe we should acquire some other data."

God whips out a laptop from under His robes and types away. In a twinkling, there are columns of figures.

"Have a look," He says, turning the screen so Ford may see. "As you can see for yourself, Mr. Ford, the latest data indicate that more men are riding my invention than are riding yours."

And as for men:

> On the Failures of Men
>
> Men have 17 parts that don't work:
>> 10 nails that don't nail
>>
>> 2 tits that don't give milk
>>
>> 2 balls that don't bounce
>>
>> 1 belly button that doesn't button
>>
>> 1 cock that won't crow
>>
>> 1 ass that won't work

While the language for both jokes is degrading in some literal ways, the humorous naming of these parts is celebrative in its own odd way. Another pun-laden joke continues with men:

> A shy woman goes to the pharmacist with some trepidation. She asks whether a particular new drug can really give her some husband some erectile assistance.
>
> "Yes," the pharmacist replies, "I can assure you that it can."
>
> "Can you get it over the counter?" she continues.
>
> Says the pharmacist, "Yes, but only if I take two."

This joke has had wide circulation because of its efficiency in a very short format and because of its clever word play. In this case, the punch line causes us to go back to the previous line, in which all seven words of the woman's speech have double meanings. (Indeed the first speech of the pharmacist can also be re-evaluated; now we know his assurance is based on personal experience.) At play also is the frankness of the pharmacist in speaking of his gigantic erection, a challenge (of sorts) to the shy woman before him, not to mention other customers who might see such a spectacular image from a healthcare professional in his place of work. The pharmacy as a whole is eroticized as well as his relationship to the woman.

Ambiguous Words, Including Ones We Don't Consider Ambiguous

Four out of five people occasionally suffer from diarrhea. The fifth person enjoys it.

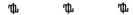

Patient: Doctor, there's something odd with me. Every time I sneeze I have an orgasm.

Doctor: That is very odd, indeed. Are you taking anything for it?

Patient: Oh heck yes, lots of fresh ground black pepper!

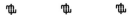

Hello! You have reached the Breast Self-Exam Hotline. For assistance, please press one now! Now press the other one!

While puns provide us with words that have two meanings, ordinary words can assume secondary and laughable meanings within a joke. In this Hotline joke, the first "one" meaning a number is replaced by a "one," which turns out to mean the other breast. With the time delay, we might call them sequential puns. The fun for the hearer/listener comes in the re-assignment of meaning to the pivotal words.

"Doctor, doctor, you must come quickly; my wife's in labor," the man yelled over the telephone.

"Is this her first child?" asked the doctor.

"No, you idiot, this is her husband!"

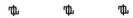

"Mr. Jones, I'm sorry to say this, but you are grossly overweight."

Mr. Jones, "I want a second opinion!"

"OK, you're stupid as well."

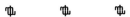

"Doctor, doctor, you must help me! I've swallowed a razorblade!"

"Oh my heavens! What have you done about it so far?"

"Well, I shaved with my electric razor."

These three jokes illustrate a conversation of A then B then A again. The first A speech is the premise, the B response builds in a reasonable direction, and the second A speech is absurd, pivoting on an ambiguity in the B response, an ambiguity inflicted by the clownish A punch line. The jokes have high energy in their short compass, and strange shifts from ordinary logic to comic logic.

The following, more extended joke uses verbal ambiguity to play on taboo subjects:

A woman is a beginner golfer; on one of her first rounds she's stung on the hand by a bee. She drives her golf cart back to the clubhouse and asks for help. An attendant calls out, "Is there a doctor in the house?"

A man at the bar stands up and says, "Yes, I'm a doctor; how can I help you?"

"This lady here," the attendant says.

"I've been stung by a bee," she says.

"Oh heck, that's too bad. Well, it probably isn't serious, but just where were you stung?"

"Between the first and the second hole."

"Hmmm. Well, the first thing I'd say is that your stance is too wide."

MEDICAL TERMS VARIOUSLY AT RISK FOR JOKING

Sometimes even the sounds of words can bring enjoyment.

A smart young doctor liked to stop at a trendy bar on his way home from work. Each day he tried a different drink. It took him almost a month to get through all the martinis and then he moved on to daiquiris. The imaginative bartender produced one variation after another, even moving on to nut flavors, almond, pistachio, walnut. The doctor enjoyed guessing what the flavor was, but one day he was totally stumped.

"Say, whatever is this flavor? I just can't make it out."

"Well, that's a hickory daiquiri, doc."

So... a social trend, a doctor, and a nursery rhyme come together just for the fun of it. The nickname "doc" is one way we seek to domesticate the physicians we trust with our lives.

Medical terminology has troubled lay people for a long time, probably for as long as there have been healers of any sort with specialized vocabularies. In the medieval world, a doctor's Latin was often fragmentary, even a sham or hoax from the lay point of view. Because medical education was often informal, almost anyone could claim to be a doctor. Indeed our modern term of derision "quack doctor" comes from the Dutch "quacksalver," or one who makes noise about salves—something akin to a snake-oil salesman or any old noisy duck. In Donizetti's opera *The Elixir of Love*, the charlatan "Doctor" Dulcamara boasts that his bottles of cheap wine can cure anything.

Today's medical terminology is a (more or less) justifiable language of a guild, an authentic jargon of professionals; nonetheless, its distinctive nature makes it a target for satire from both outsiders and insiders. Bernard J. Freedman's delightful book *Just a Word, Doctor* includes some eighty short essays originally published in the *British Medical Journal.* These play with etymology, medical history, cross-cultural usages, and more; Dr. Freedman whimsically mixes humor and lexicography, showing that words have many strange dimensions.[4]

Some jokes are largely playful, although they still attempt to domesticate medical language, even the simplest of medical terms.

A window (hard to picture, but never mind) goes to the see a doctor and complains that it's experiencing several panes.

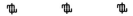

Advertising sign in a psychiatrist's window: Satisfaction guaranteed or your mania back.

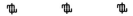

How do crazy people walk through the forest? They take the psychopath.

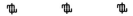

A man calls into work sick one day and says, "Boss, I don't think I'm going to make it into the office today. I'm sick."

The suspicious boss asks, "Oh yeah? Just what do you have?"

The man replies, "I'm afraid I have anal glaucoma."

"Anal glaucoma? What the hell is that?"

"It means I just can't see my ass coming in to work today."

Another thematically similar play on words is this parody of a medical definition:

Optical rectosis: the condition of having a shitty outlook on life.

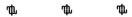

A Czechoslovakian man felt his eyesight was growing steadily worse, so that it was time to visit an optometrist. The doctor set him 20 feet away from a standard eye chart with the large letters at the top and the progressively smaller ones below.

"Can you read this?" the doctor said, indicating the letters:

CRXSNKXZY.

"Read it? Heck, I know the man."

And from the doctor's side:

A doctor examines a patient, takes an exhaustive history, does every imaginable lab test, every imaginable imaging modality, and finally—with the help of the Internet—reaches a diagnosis.

Returning to the examining room, the doctor tells the patient: "You have a disease so rare, I haven't a clue how to pronounce it."

Some jokes about terminology pivot on patients who are unable to understand medical concepts. Their stupidity makes them scapegoats, persons we reject from the human family.

Here is a pair of jokes cast in letter form, presumably from non-compos-mentis correspondents:

Dear Doctor,

My wife and I are both sterile, certainly a disturbing condition. Is there any chance that we might pass this trait along to our children?

⚕   ⚕   ⚕

Dear Doctor,

My husband and I have two lovely children and are considering having a third. But I just read that every third child born today is Chinese. Since we are both of Norwegian descent, do you think we should take such a risk?

The following joke combines a medical pun with yet another anal taboo.

Emergency Restaurant Intervention

Two nurses are having lunch at a café when a man at a nearby table staggers from his table, clutching his throat. His eyes bug out; his face is bright red.

"Oh damn," one nurse says. "I think it's my turn."

She puts down her napkin, jumps up, and knocks the man to the floor. She undoes his belt buckle, flips him over, and pulls down his pants and undershorts. When she licks up his ass groove with her tongue, he shudders and spits up a gob of meat. His color and breathing return to normal.

"My God, you've saved my life, young woman! How can I ever thank you?" he says.

"Yeah, sure, fine, whatever," the nurse says, waving him away.

She goes back to her table, soaks her napkin in her water glass, and wipes off her tongue.

She tells her companion, "I just hate doing the Hind Lick Maneuver."

There's also a cowboy version of this joke:

A woman sitting at a restaurant in a small Texas town suddenly begins to make terrible choking sounds while eating an armadillo omelet. Two cowboys at a neighboring table look over in alarm and note her distress.

"Well, kin yuh swaller?" asks one.

She shakes her head in the negative.

"Kin yuh breathe okie dokie?" asks the other.

Now turning quite red, her eyes bugged out, she signals no and points to her throat. She rises from her table, staggering.

At that news, the first cowboy walks over to her, lifts up the back of her skirt, and yanks down her underpants. He kneels behind her then runs his tongue up her behind.

She experiences a convulsion that produces a tremendous cough, and some indeterminate portion of an armadillo flies out of her mouth and across the room. She draws in an unobstructed breath and smiles her thanks to the cowboy, who tips his hat and swaggers his way back to his seat.

His partner says, "Well, now, I surely have heard of the Hind Lick Maneuver, but I reckon that's the very first time I've ever seen it done!"

The Heimlich maneuver is, of course, well known, publicized on posters in restaurant kitchens and in mass media for years. Besides the obvious pun worked in these two jokes, the characters are of opposites sexes in each joke, suggesting some heterosexual eroticism, even breaking taboos against anal sex. The sexual implications combined with the life-and-death meaning of choking provides good tension which is relieved by the unexpected pun and an image of convulsion and expulsion that has resonances with orgasm. The Texas version uses an approximation of regional dialect to satirize the supposed stupidity of country people, although here, of course, the cowboy is actually the hero of the story.

In the next joke, a doctor willfully misuses his power and misnames (perhaps ethically) a diagnosis:

A 70-year-old woman went to a clinic with a terrible and long-lasting case of hiccups. By chance, there was a new doctor who saw her.

"Yes, you do have quite a case of hiccups," he said. "But I think you have a more serious problem: you are pregnant."

The woman screamed and ran out of the exam room and down the hall, still screaming. The senior doctor intercepted her, calmed her, and took her to another room, where he heard the whole story. He asked her to wait a moment while he confronted the new doctor.

"What the hell do you mean, shocking Mrs. Stevens like that? She has three grown children and five grandchildren, and you tell her she's pregnant?"

Said the young doctor, "But does she still have hiccups?"

Occasionally an ambiguous phrase can be a tautology, a verbal construct that is self-reflexive without reference to the outside world.

A patient says, "Doctor, I don't feel well."

The doctor says, "Have you had this before?"

The patient says, "Yes, I have."

And the doctor says, "We'll, I'm afraid you've got it again."

This cynical little joke expresses our fear that doctors don't really know what they're talking about and that the doctor-patient encounter is a sham. In this case, the doctor is a parody of the active listener, putting all meanings back on the patient while providing none of his own. Thus there's a suggestion of blaming the patient for his or her own malaise. The pronouns with nonexistent referents ("this," "it") keep the patient in the same uncertainty he or she experienced before seeking medical help.

By contrast, one of the comforting features of medical care is the pronouncement of a diagnosis, literally something that is "known" by the physician, recognized as a disease that people do get, so that we feel relief when we hear a diagnosis. (I'm speaking now of relatively simple diseases and injuries here, but even a serious diagnosis can provide relief from uncertainty.) A diagnosis for an easily treated disease is especially comforting, since patients can stop worrying about more serious conditions and proceed to treatment. A diagnosis partakes of the Word Magic discussed earlier; when the doctor gives us a diagnosis, we feel we have control over something that has been troubling our bodies and, therefore, our minds. We are no longer an isolated, unique absurdity.

MALAPROPISMS AND OTHER RIDICULOUS LINGUISTIC MISTAKES

Mrs. Malaprop is a character in Sheridan's *The Rivals*, a comic play of 1775. She uses words incorrectly, words that sound like other words, for example "an allegory by the banks of the Nile." Her last name has the meaning, in French, of "not appropriate." The late (and most entertaining) comedian George Carlin was famous for his short formulations that show irrational features of our language. Some of his Carlinisms have medical subjects: "If athletes get athlete's foot, do astronauts get mistletoe?" and "If blind people wear dark glasses, why don't deaf people wear earmuffs?"

There are several versions of the following joke, all punishing the main character for his lack of linguistic clarity:

A man goes to his doctor to request castration. The doctor says this is a very serious request and sends him away to think it all over. A week later he's back, saying he's made up his mind. The doctor admits him to the hospital and removes the man's testicles. Recovering in his hospital room, he asks the man in the next bed what he's in for.

"Oh, nothing much; I came in to be circumcised."

"Oh, son of a bitch! That's the word I meant!"

The two confused words have three syllables, both start with "c," and both have Latin roots. We may laugh at this man's confusion (and appropriate punishment), but probably all of us have confused medical terms at some time or another (for example some drugs, in brand and/or generic names).

In one rare case, a patient can't remember the common word:

A man walks into the drug store and asks for acetylsalicylic acid.

"Surely you mean aspirin," the druggist replies.

"Oh yeah," the man says. "I can never remember that word."

Short Satiric Structures

In the following chapters, we'll look at parodies of longer verbal structures, but here we can look at some word play that parodies advertising signs.

Medical Signs

On the maternity room door: PUSH, PUSH, PUSH

In the vet's waiting room: SIT! STAY!!

At the podiatrist's: TIME WOUNDS ALL HEELS.

At the optometrist's: IF YOU DON'T SEE WHAT YOU'RE LOOKING FOR, YOU'RE IN THE RIGHT PLACE.

At the proctologist's: TO EXPEDITE YOUR VISIT, PLEASE BACK IN.

In front of the funeral home: DRIVE CAREFULLY: WE'LL WAIT.

At the gynecologist's office: AT YOUR CERVIX, MADAM; DILATED TO MEET YOU.

The gynecologist's sign (or supposed greeting) has been around for at least fifty years; I first heard it from my father in the 1950s. It owes its durability to the two puns and to the psychodynamic of (presumed) male intimacy to a woman who has opened (or allowed to be opened) her private (taboo) parts willingly. There's an oddity in suggesting that the doctor is "dilated," since dilation in the medical sense refers to the enlargement of the os (mouth) of the cervix (neck of the womb) during labor for childbirth, although the doctor, the joke suggests, may be delighted to be looking at her genitals.

Another short structure that has been satirized is the "health hint" found in magazines and newspapers. Here are a few that have circulated on the Internet:

> For a toothache, smash your thumb with a hammer so you'll forget about the toothache.

> High blood pressure? No problem! Cut yourself and bleed for a while. It's probably a good idea to use a timer.

> If you are choking on an ice cube, stay calm. Pour some boiling water down your throat to remove the obstruction.

> For a bad cough, take a large dose of laxatives so that you'll be afraid to cough.

IN SUMMARY

Although puns and other plays on words seem to criticize language by showing how inexact it is, they also celebrate it as an artistic medium because of its sounds, its nuances, its levels of meaning and emotion, and, above all, its ambiguous, quicksilver nature. Language opens up another world of meaning only partially attached to the real world or what we believe to be the real world. When language is free from the usual demands of exactitude, logic, and seriousness, it can allow our imaginations to relax, expand, and play. An appropriate motto for the literary comedian and punster could be this: Fight absurdity, chaos, and evil with silly language! Such language suggests that we have freedom—freedom to misuse language, to point out absurdities, and to be silly even for no ordinary good purpose. And "silly," we may recall, once had the sense of innocence; one Christmas carol refers to "silly sheep." Indeed, the word "silly" comes from Old English *saelig*, meaning "happy" or "blessed," as in the modern German "selig." Perhaps language play is a reverential, even priestly act. When people exchange puns, limericks, and other jokes that emphasize the irrational features of language, they form comic communities that seek happiness, social solidarity, and emotional re-evaluations of subjects that make us nervous or even frighten us. To be in the Green World of comedy is to dwell, however temporarily, in a blessed, free community.

English is especially good for language play because of its very large vocabulary, its high idiomatic content (as in "putting the dog down"), and its wide range of meanings from formal medical terminology to dirty words. Indeed the English language itself may have its own risks, if the following joke is to be believed:

The Dangers of Speaking English

Anthropologists have studied language and health, concluding that:

1. The Japanese eat very little fat and suffer fewer heart attacks than Americans.

2. The Mexicans eat a lot of fat and suffer fewer heart attacks than Americans.

3. The Chinese drink very little red wine and suffer fewer heart attacks than Americans.

4. The Italians drink a lot of red wine and suffer fewer heart attacks than Americans.

5. The Germans drink a lot of beer and eat lots of sausages and fats and suffer fewer heart attacks than Americans.

Therefore, you should eat and drink anything you wish, because it's not the food and drink that kill you but speaking English.

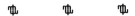

There's a warning attributed to Mark Twain: "Be careful reading health books. You may die of a misprint."

Finally—as in the last salvo of fireworks at a July 4th celebration—here is a punful contribution from our British friends:

A Panel of Doctors

When a panel of doctors was asked to vote on adding a new wing to their hospital, the Allergists voted to scratch it and the Dermatologists advised no rash moves. The Gastroenterologists had a gut feeling about it, but the Neurologists thought the administration had a lot of nerve, and the Obstetricians stated they were all labouring under a misconception. The Ophthalmologists considered the idea short-sighted; the Pathologists yelled, "Over my dead body!" while the Pediatricians said, "Grow up!" The Psychiatrists thought the whole idea was madness; the Surgeons decided to wash their hands of the whole thing, and the Radiologists could see right through it. The Internists thought it was a bitter pill to swallow, but the Plastic Surgeons said, "This puts a whole new face on the matter." The Podiatrists thought it was a step forward, but the Urologists felt the scheme wouldn't hold water. The Anesthesiologists thought the whole idea was a gas, and the Cardiologists didn't have the heart to say no. And in the end, the Proctologists said, "Forward the issue to some asshole who wouldn't give a shit."

Chapter Six

Imagine That!

Images of the Regrettably Mechanical Body

The Woman In A Halo Brace At Christmas Time

ONE CHRISTMAS SEASON, I saw a woman in a wheelchair being pushed down a hospital hall; she was wearing a halo brace, a metal circle that fits like a halo around the top of the head. Such a brace stabilizes a patient's neck following an injury and/or surgery. This circle doesn't simply "fit," however; it's actually pinned to the skull with screws, which typically cause headaches at first. The halo brace differs from a halo in a religious painting because it has metal columns that descend vertically, two at the side of the face, and sometimes two to the rear of the head. These columns end up in a collar that rests on the collarbones and shoulders of the patient or a plastic vest that goes round the patient's torso. Either way, the brace immobilizes the neck and head for twelve weeks or more. One provider of the braces says that they provide "complete fixation" of the head. It is hard to imagine a more mechanical phrase than that.

The brace makes many ordinary activities very awkward: washing hair, eating, getting dressed, even reading; the patient can't drive a car. Since the brace weighs about seven pounds, balance is changed and falls are a danger. Patients complain that putting eight to ten pins in their skulls is painful, that sleeping in the device is difficult, that they feel like Frankenstein's monster, and so on. As awkward as the brace is, it is a treatment preferred over weeks or months of bed rest that can be boring and debilitating, and many patients are grateful to avoid a body cast or surgery.

This woman's halo brace was unusual: woven into it were red ribbons, green ivy, some tiny ornaments, and mistletoe. She was a mobile Christmas tree or maybe a holly wreath, given the similar circles. Not only did she call attention to her mechanical device, but she also domesticated it by bringing it into her version of the Green World. Like signatures or expressions of "Get well soon" written on a cast, her decorations advertised her own acceptance and redefinition of the brace. In domesticating her brace, she advertised her wit and public statement of her positive attitude about it. Since mistletoe is commonly hung in doorways of houses, her brace was linked to the concept of home. Her decorated brace suggested that she was still participating in the social give and take of a healthy person. Since custom allows people to kiss under mistletoe, she was symbolically saying that she was available for kissing every minute of every day, no matter where she was. It's likely that she had other people do much of the decorating, perhaps supportive family and friends who will further assist her during the weeks or months she wears the halo brace.

The halo brace looks medieval, a kind of mobile prison that may make us think of the Man in the Iron Mask or even chastity belts (as in John Hawkes' novel *Blood Oranges*). Like an iron lung, a body cast, or traction setups in a hospital bed, the brace appears to take over the living person mechanically. (Other imprisonments are pharmaceutical, as in a drug-induced coma for a burn patient). People may stare at a halo brace in public, unused to seeing this odd contraption; sometimes they'll look quickly away, an avoidance ritual. Our decorated woman, however, invited looking and reflection on the strange dialectic she had created between the medical and the domestic.

We can speculate further on other features. The name of this device, "halo brace," has an attractive vowel harmony of the matching "a" sounds. "Halo," of course, suggests a kind of holiness, an emanation of energy around a person of deep spirituality, in ironic contrast to intractable metal. "Halo brace" is a bold euphemism, making light of an imprisoning structure but perhaps paying homage to a miracle of design that can save a person not only from surgery but also from paralysis.

To be "at home" with a halo brace (or an injury or an illness, even a terminal illness) is to bring it within a structure of values and emotions that tame it and bring it into a comfortable relationship, if not outright control. In Yiddish, a "haimisher mensch," is someone you feel comfortable with. "Haimish" is a variant of the German, "heimisch," which relates to "heim" or "home." The synonyms in one German-English dictionary are instructive about the localized Green Worlds that patients may try to create around illness: homey, native, endemic, homelike, domestic, regional, indigenous. "Heimish" is thus related to the earth and nature as well as to the people we choose to affiliate with.

As I discussed the Christmas halo brace with a Rehab nurse years later, she recalled a patient who had a similar brace. His version of humor to domesticate his brace was quite different: he'd roam the halls of the Rehab unit and suddenly jump out to surprise people. He'd produce a bizarre laugh and announce that he was an alien from another planet. This man chose the highly energized role of a joker. By contrast, the woman with Christmas decorations chose more of a clowning, domestic role.

Years ago, I sprained my ankle and spent four weeks in a fiberglass cast. The only place I didn't feel that I was an anomaly was in the waiting room of my orthopedic surgeon, where the majority of people had casts; the others were friends and family who accepted our appearances and implied histories. Although initially strangers, we freely exchanged information about our injuries, the absurdity of our accidents and/ or our stupidity, the medical treatment, and, of course, how long the carapace-like casts were to stay on our bodies. Equally outsiders to healthy America, we made our own comic community.

When our mental lives are full, we often pay little attention to our bodies. When we focus on a conversation, for example, we forget the bodies that make it possible. Indeed, modern cultures are so dominated by radio, TV, cell phones, and all the intensities of urban life that we live in our heads much of the time. If we walk by a store window, however, we see the reflection of the front or sides of our body. If we use a hand mirror, we can see every part, often making judgments about how well or poorly we appear.

Furthermore, all of our body reports to our consciousness via sensory nerves. If we step on a child's toy in the dark, our foot has some immediate news for us. If there's gas in our lower bowel, nerves tell us about it, and we have to make plans. If we take out some clothes from last winter and find that they don't fit, we pat our bellies, feel our waists, and wonder just what happened here? For better or worse, we live in our bodies, bodies that can bring us much pleasure or much pain, bodies that we feel comfortable with, that we can criticize, or even ignore.

Clearly we have conflicting and contradictory attitudes about our bodies. On the one hand, we take pleasure in the movement of our bodies as we dance or play sports. We enjoy a hike that takes us to vistas of scenery. We enjoy laughter, close contact with loved ones, and all the ways sensuous pleasures come to us, such as good food and drink with all the attendant sights, smells, tastes, and textures.

But our brains and social norms yearn for perfection. Popular magazines have stories about "body image," our personal perception of how our bodies appear to others and to ourselves. Such interest can be reasonable and normal, or it can be an illness, an obsession known as "body dysmorphic disorder," a psychological illness characterized by obsessive concern about the appearance of the body. Perceptions of our bodies can be anywhere on a range of normalcy, narcissism, or pathology.

Let's turn now to the oral tradition to see other ways of playing with images of the human body.

From The World of Jokes

A couple had been debating the purchase of a new auto for weeks. He wanted a new truck. She wanted a fast little sports-like car so she could zip through traffic around town. He would probably have settled on any beat-up old truck, but everything she seemed to like was far out of their price range.

"Look!" she said. "I want something that goes from 0 to 200 in 4 seconds or less. And my birthday is coming up. You could surprise me."

For her birthday, he bought her a brand new bathroom scale.

Our bodies have weight, volume, texture, shape, size, color, and other attributes of solids, and we sense the ironic distance between perfect bodies and the actual ones we inhabit. Humor is a typical way of dealing with such disparities, and the use of literary imagery is a powerful way of representing our fears and aversions about the human body. The vengeful husband in the joke above not only denies his wife's wish for a sports car, but he insults her by giving her a scale that could assess her avoirdupois up to 200 pounds.

Not only do our bodies exist in space, they clearly exist in time; our bodies that grow older year by year, decade by decade, and ultimately fall apart after death. As we mature from childhood we watch our bodies change, often with some nervousness about whether we are the right size and shape, whether we look right compared to our peers, or how we compare with images in magazines, on TV, or the movies. As we come into sexual maturity, we are concerned about our attractiveness; will anyone find us attractive? Consciously and unconsciously, we learn cues for sexual attraction. Some of these (styles in clothing, hair, makeup) are socially created and change rapidly from decade to decade. Other cues are millennia old, probably with instinctual, even genetic roots; we prize symmetry of bodies and faces, athletic looks, good skin, clear eyes, and strong, even teeth, all markers of health and evolutionary success; a potential partner with these qualities should produce healthy and successful children who can help us in our old age—should we be lucky enough to reach it—and who can create the next generations.

As we age, however, we typically lose flexibility, strength, sexual prowess, and endurance. These losses become exaggerated when we are ill; if we regain our health, we feel gratitude in recapturing them. If there are permanent losses, we must deal with them. Decline with advancing age is a harbinger of death, which we fear because of instinct and cultural interpretation. While mortality per se is not curable, there are ways to heal it, that is, to find understanding and even acceptance.

Clearly there's a lot tied up in how we live in our bodies, what we want from them, what we're nervous about, or what we downright fear. Given this welter of emotions and conflicting ideas, it's no surprise that we yearn to fight irrationality with irrationality, calling on humor to help us represent and interpret our dilemmas and also to provide joking rituals that assure us that we aren't alone in our neuroses about our bodies.

The Powers of Imagery

Humor is all too glad to enlist the resources of imagery, that is, language that appeals to the senses, notably the classic five senses. In the rest of this chapter, we'll look at (1) these five senses, then (2) parts of bodies, and last (3) shape-shifting through plastic surgery.

Let's look at four jokes that emphasize visual imagery and thereby engage our visual imaginations.

Five surgeons are discussing who makes the best patients to operate on. The first surgeon says, "I really like to see accountants on my operating table, because when you open them up, everything inside is numbered."

"That's helpful," replied the second, "but my favorite are actually electricians; everything in them is color coded."

"In my book," said the third, "it's librarians who are by far the easiest: everything in them is in alphabetical order."

The fourth surgeon said, "For me, construction workers are the most convenient, not simply because of how orderly they're put together, but even more because they understand if you have a few parts left over in the end and if the job takes longer than you said it would."

The last surgeon couldn't wait any longer. "All of you are nuts. The easiest persons in the universe to work on are politicians: they have no guts, no balls, no heart, no spine, and no brain. Also, the head and the ass are interchangeable."

In this joke, we consider the visual images of the electricians' color-coded body parts. As we read or hear this joke, our minds may flash on images we have seen of electrical equipment or schematic drawings, even the back of a VCR/TV setup that we puzzled over. This process, of course, is the activity of our imagination, as we recall and manipulate images to create some kind of order. The first three surgeons are somewhat parallel in their images of organization; the fourth expands into the world of construction and the fifth adds a satiric dimension about politicians. This joke suggests that even if we are limited in our bodies, our imaginations can be wonderfully free.

A woman goes to see a sex therapist.

"My husband," she reports, "always falls asleep with his erect penis still inside me."

"Well, that might be nice. But you're here for some reason. Is there a problem?" the therapist asks.

"Why yes, in fact: he walks in his sleep."

We read the simple, monosyllabic words of the punch line, then take a moment to create our own personal images of how the copulating couple just might make their way around their darkened house, without benefit of clothes, linked by his penis, which is burdened by much of her weight, minus whatever load she has taken with her arms and hands or maybe chin on his shoulder—well, of course, it's ridiculous and physically impossible. We laugh at the image and at the improbability of the conversation with a therapist. (Does he or she immediately burst out in laughter?) The entire medical interview is a parody of what a therapeutic conversation might be and hinges on the punch line which fires our imagination to create the visual images of this unusual couple.

A similar joke is this:

A woman goes to the doctor and complains of knee pains. He examines them and finds that they are indeed sore but with no apparent structural reason for injury.

"Are you sure you've told me everything?"

"Well," says she. "Not quite. My husband and I have sex doggy style every night."

"Bingo," says the doctor. "We can solve this right away: there are plenty of other positions for intercourse."

She says, "Not if I'm going to watch TV."

The brief little story engages our imaginations to picture the scene and the characters' relationship, which apparently includes her disinterest in sex with her husband.

An overbearing surgeon has been admitted as a patient. Noisy and demanding, he is a trial to all the nurses attending him. After several younger nurses visit him (some departing in tears), a senior nurse enters his room and orders him to turn over so that his temperature can be taken.

"I'll do no such thing!" he bellows.

"I'd strongly advise it, doctor, or you won't receive the treatment that will get you discharged from here."

Grudgingly he complies, and she inserts a thermometer (he thinks) into his anus and leaves the room. When she doesn't come back for several minutes, he presses the call button. Then he yells. Another nurse enters the room and bursts into raucous laughter.

"What's so funny?" he demands.

She replies, "Well, doctor, it's just that I've never seen a temperature being taken with an Easter lily."

Here, the visual impact occurs twice, once within the story itself and again in our minds as we imagine the scene. The senior nurse has punished the doctor for his churlish behavior through a visual pun, the substitution of the lily for the thermometer, a flower that suggests women's culture, springtime, Easter, and many healthy, nonmedical milieus. Furthermore, her anal insertion of this lily has resonances with flowers arising from dirt, even fecal matter. A more brutal resonance, of course, is rape, here performed by a woman in order to demean a man. Fortunately, the next nurse who sees the lily in situ feels not horror but hilarity, and we are invited to laugh with her...and against the scapegoated doctor. There are also dynamics of revenge between lily-wielding nurse and crabby doctor, between female and male, between a "normal person" and a humour character (choleric, in this case).

A morally similar joke punishes a professional from the funeral trade:

An embalmer was preparing the body of one Mr. Gondorf, when he found that Mr. Gondorf had a remarkably thick and long penis, in fact the largest he had ever observed. He marveled at this prodigy but felt ethical constraints about sharing this information with anyone. The knowledge weighed on him, however, to the extent that he felt he could share it with the one person he trusted most. Accordingly, he took a scalpel and removed the organ, carrying it home in his lunchbox. That night, at dinner, he opened the lunchbox and held up the item, about to explain about it, when his wife burst out, "Oh my God, Gondorf is dead!"

This joke displays the trope of the trickster tricked, an ancient theme. The unethical embalmer receives poetic justice through his wife's unfaithfulness, and the pivotal portion of the mutilated Gondorf has its revenge in the embalmer's own home.

In our mind's eye, we imagine, we see the lunch-boxed penis, the buttocked lily, the copulating couple near a TV, the nocturnal couple in peripatetic carnal embrace, and the color-coded entrails.

WHAT DID HENRI BERGSON SAY ABOUT PHYSICAL HUMOR?

Henri Bergson (1859-1941) was a French philosopher who wrote a long, long treatise on humor, entitled *Le rire: Essai sur la signification du comique* (1913; *Laughter: An Essay on the Meaning of the Comic*). Being a philosopher, Bergson went on at considerable length about two simple but powerful ideas. First, the stiffness (*raideur*) of the humor body is in itself laughable because it suggests stiffness of character, which is anti-social. So the cartoon cliché of a man slipping on a banana peel and falling—and all other pratfalls—is funny because his stiffness is being loosened up. The woman with the halo brace transformed her mechanical entrapment to an image of festive energy. Second, the human body is organic and plastic ordinarily, but humorous when it acts like a machine in, say, mechanical materials with no minds, imaginations, or freedom. The great comics on film such as Charlie Chaplin and Jacques Tati were masters of physical humor which appeared both stiff and mechanical.

Mechanical stiffness (along with some puns) is illustrated in this joke:

A man slowly boarding a bus held up the line of people behind him. He turned and offered this apology to the man just behind him: "You'll have to excuse me for being so slow; I'm a little stiff from rowing."

To which the man replied, "Oh, that's OK, and my name's Schultz, from Cleveland."

And from a medical setting:

Mr. Jones goes to visit his 90-year-old father in a nursing home.

"How they treating you, Pops?"

"Right good, son. Right good."

"Food OK?"

"Yeah, you bet."

"Nurses nice?"

"They're fine. Nice gals."

"Are you sleeping OK?"

"Dandy. Eight hours straight through. About 9:30 they bring me a cup of hot chocolate and that new stuff, Viagra."

"Viagra? Are you sure?"

"Yep. And I sleep good!"

Mr. Jones is alarmed but hides his feelings until the visit is over. He then goes to the medical director and says, "You want to hear something funny? My dad thinks you're giving him Viagra every night!"

"Oh, but it's true...along with the hot chocolate."

"What? Whatever for?"

"Well, the milk and the chocolate help him sleep, and the Viagra stops him from rolling out of bed."

There's a similar joke about Viagra given for bad sunburn, so that sheets no longer touch the man.

The following joke gives a cross-profession look at mechanics:

Dr. White, a surgeon, has taken his BMW into the dealership for some work. When he arrives to pick, it up a mechanic recognizes him and calls him over.

"Look at this," he says, gesturing to the engine compartment of another fine sports car. "I do all the stuff you do, work on the insides, refine the tuning, clean out grease and junk, and make it run like new. So how come you get huge dollars and I'm living paycheck to paycheck?"

Dr. White asks, "Yes, but can you do all that while the motor is running?"

Another (and rather strange) joke goes like this:

An OB/GYN is bored with his profession and takes a class at a community college in auto mechanics. For the final exam, all the students are to dissemble an engine.

The instructor is pleased that all students pass the test but gives the doctor extra points because he took the engine apart through the muffler.

LARGER AND SMALLER

As we view our own bodies and assess their shortcomings, we are delighted to consider exaggerated images of abnormality that go well beyond our own personal dilemmas. Images of gigantism, miniaturization, bizarre changes in shape, and so on give us a very large circle of imaginative possibility, helping us focus our small variations within a smaller circle that we can consider normal or, in the medical phrase, "within normal limits."

A woman who happened to be a midget went to her doctor's office on a rainy day and explained her problem: "You know, doc, every time it rains like this I have pain in my crotch."

"Well, that's unusual, but hop up on the table and let's see what the problem is. Um, well, I guess I'd better get a chair, so you can climb up."

She does so, and he says, "I think I can help you out." He works on her a while, then says, "I think we have a solution. Hop down—er, use the chair—and tell me how you feel."

She does so and says, "Golly, you solved it. What did you do?"

"I cut two inches off the top of your galoshes."

Sometimes imagery wildly changes the size of ordinary objects.

While sleeping one day on a sofa, a man snores with his mouth open. A curious mouse investigates this aperture and falls in. The man wakes up, coughing terribly. His wife rushes in and observes his distress.

She calls the doctor: "Doctor, doctor, you must help us! My husband has swallowed a mouse and is coughing and thrashing. His face is red and he's desperate!"

"I'll be right over, but meanwhile, get the smelliest cheese you have in the house and wave it over your husband's mouth in order to entice the mouse to come out!"

The doctor arrives and sees the man sprawled out on the floor. His wife is kneeling by him; her arm is moving.

Ah, this is good, the doctor thinks. But then he sees that she is holding smoked herring, not cheese.

"Oh no! I distinctly said cheese!" he cries out.

"I know, I know," replies the wife, "but first I've got to get the damn cat out of him!"

Clearly we're in the land of the tall-tale (or tail), where fantasy creates scenes that are physically impossible but surprising and entertaining. This is the world of cartoons, science fiction, mythological narrative, even supernatural scripture. In the world of comedy, we can enjoy the plastic nature of our material bodies; here, our general fear of having something bad in our mouths is gigantized through the image of the cat. We may further enjoy the woman's independence in her problem-solving skills and her variation on the doctor's orders.

Sometimes imagery recontexts ordinary things.

A prankster laid down glue on a toilet seat at a store, and unsuspecting Mr. Jones sat on it and was held fast. He tried to free himself, but to no avail. He called for help. Store employees sympathized and apologized, but they could do nothing to free him. They called the paramedics.

The paramedics arrived, sympathized, but also could not free Mr. Jones from the toilet seat. The best they could do was to unbolt the seat from the toilet and transport him to an Emergency Room.

When the doctor saw the situation, he said, "Over the years I've seen a lot of these, but I believe this is the first time I've seen one framed."

Given his time and place, Prof. Bergson did not write about feces and urine, but he should have. The excremental images of scatological humor are, of course, breakings of taboo, allowing us to admit that they exist and to bring humor to them for rituals of laughter, but they are also clearly part of the physical workings of our bodies. In the curmudgeonly surgeon joke, the image of the flower blossoming out of his posterior provides us with high comedy.

Sometimes the physical nature of the body complicates another character's actions.

Jim and Edna were both patients in a mental hospital. One day while they were walking past the hospital swimming pool, Jim suddenly jumped into the deep end. He sank to the bottom of the pool and stayed there. Edna promptly jumped in after him. She swam to the bottom and pulled Jim out.

When the Head Nurse Director became aware of Edna's heroic act, she immediately ordered Edna to be discharged from the hospital, considering her now to be mentally stable.

When she went to tell Edna the news she said, "Edna, I have good news and bad news. The good news is you're being discharged. Since you were able to rationally respond to a crisis by jumping in and saving the life of another patient, I have concluded that your act displays sound mindedness. The bad news is that Jim, the patient you saved, hanged himself with his bathrobe belt in the bathroom right after you saved him. I am so sorry, but I must tell you that he's dead."

Edna replied, "Oh, heck, I know that, and he didn't hang himself. I put him there to dry. How soon can I go home?"

Compared to other topics, there are fewer jokes dealing with mental deficits.

PROTESTS AGAINST MEDICAL MECHANIZATION

As we all know, the medical encounter can leave us feeling like a piece of meat, especially when medical machines are involved. The following script, widely disseminated on the Internet, is a parody of medical instructions; the parody is sarcastic, a rebellion against the demeaning experience of the mammogram.

How To Prepare For Your Mammogram

While some women are nervous about their first mammogram, there is really no need for such concern. The following three simple exercises should help you feel prepared, confident, and entirely ready for the experience. These exercises are simple; they need no fancy equipment. You can do them in the privacy of your own home. Just a few minutes a day for 10-14 days before your exam should make everything go smoothly.

Exercise #1

Having bared your chest, open your refrigerator door and insert one breast between the door and the main cabinet. Have your husband or any other large person push the door as shut as possible and lean upon it. Hold for five seconds and repeat with the other breast.

Exercise #2

Go to your garage at 5:00 a.m. when the cement floor should be the coldest. (If you do not have such a garage, ask to use a friend's or, even better, a stranger's.) Remove all clothing and lie comfortably on the floor with one breast wedged under the rear tire. Have a friend back the car over the breast for optimal flattening and chilling. Spin around and repeat with other breast. Avoid inhaling exhaust fumes.

Exercise #3

Freeze two metal bookends overnight. Bare your chest. Invite a total stranger into the room. Ask him (males preferred) to press your breast between the bookends as hard as possible. Make a date with him to do this again in one year.

Refrigerator, car, bookends—all mechanical, metallic, and cold—are adversaries to the warm, sensitive breast, and the imagery is, of course, exaggerated to absurdity. The comic catharsis is, we hope, in the naming of the unpleasant, sensual features of an actual mammogram (pressure, coldness, impersonality, breaches of modesty). The underlying fears of finding a lump, especially a cancerous one, are also indirectly expelled through laughter and a sense of solidarity with other women who also do not enjoy the procedure.

Readers of Dave Barry may recall a column about his colonoscopy; it makes similarly outlandish comparisons about the body being assailed by a mechanical, medical device.

Caregivers can also be satirized because they treat a patient mechanically.

Charles goes to visit his father in a nursing home. Dad is sitting up in a wheelchair.

"How are they treating you, Dad?"

"Oh, fine, fine." At this point, Dad leans over to his right. A nurse rushes over and straightens him up.

"The food's OK."

"The nurses kind to you?"

"Oh yeah, sure." At this point, Dad leans over to his left. A nurse rushes over and straightens him up.

"Warm enough?"

"Yeah, you bet." At this point, Dad leans over to his right. A nurse rushes over and straightens him up.

Charles is suspicious that he's not getting the whole story.

"Well, is there anything that bothers you?"

"Um, there is just one thing."

"Well, what is it?"

"Lean closer."

Charles does so.

"They won't let me fart!"

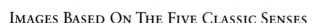

IMAGES BASED ON THE FIVE CLASSIC SENSES

Imagery that is based on our senses have exploited our classic five, although not equally. (Other senses, such as balance, temperature, proprioception, and pain are equally important to our lives but not as recognized culturally as part of the classic five and therefore not typically subjects for jokes.)

THE PRIMACY OF SEEING

We've mentioned that humans gain much of their information about the world through sight; three of our twelve cranial nerves are connected to our eyes. In particular, we assess other people visually, both consciously and unconsciously. Scientists have discovered microexpressions of the face that we perceive although unaware that we are doing so. More consciously, we see features in other persons such as height, muscularity, fat content, skin, posture, and more. At a primal level we assess whether they are friends or enemies (Could he beat me up?). In our search for sexual partners we look for symmetry and general vitality. Healthy people are attractive to us—or possible competitors.

Unhealthy people set off alarms; we wonder whether we should be around them; are they contagious? Such automatic assessments and reactions are probably the result of millennia of evolution. We quickly notice signs of illness or debility. These include limping, facial tics, an eye that wanders, and unhealthy skin. When there are mechanical aids—wheelchairs, walkers, canes, bandages, prostheses—we notice these right away and interpret from there. As children, we are taught not to stare at any of these signs, but our eyes still stay alert to them, and we may use humor to break taboos and present physical abnormality in the safe world of jokes.

One of the places where physical abnormality is seen, noticed, and commented upon is, of course, the doctor's office. Here our weakness may be shared; here privacy may be abridged.

A man walks into the doctor's office. He has a carrot up his nose, a cucumber in his right ear, and a banana in his other ear.

"Doc, I don't feel good. Whatever do you think is wrong with me?

The doctor takes a careful look and says, "You know, I just don't think you are eating *properly*.

🙂   🙂   🙂

A man goes to see his psychiatrist. When he enters the office, the psychiatrist does a double take because the man is wearing nothing but a layer of plastic wrap all around his body.

"Well, what do you think of this, doctor?" asks the man.

"Hm," replies the doctor. "I can clearly see your [you're] nuts."

This joke goes to a physical extreme beyond the human body:

Operating Room nurse: "Doctor, you mustn't cut so deep!"

"And why not?"

"That's the fourth operating table you've ruined this week!"

In this joke, patients have disappeared entirely; we can only imagine that they were sliced clear through.

The next joke uses two men on the street as observers:

Sister Mary was visiting hospital patients when her car ran out of gas. As luck would have it, a gas station was just a block away. She walked to the station to borrow a gas can and buy some gas. The attendant told her the only gas can he owned had just been loaned out, but she could wait until it was returned. Since the nun was on the way to see a patient, she decided not to wait and walked to the nearby hospital.

While talking to the patient, she looked for something she could fill with gas and spotted a bedpan. Always resourceful, she carried the bedpan to the station, filled it with gas, and carried the full bedpan back to her car.

As she was pouring the gas into her tank two men watched from across the street. One of them turned to the other and said, "If it starts, I'm turning Catholic."

SEEING IN THE MIND'S EYE

Sometimes the imagery emphasizes representations in the characters' minds. Some jokes have variations on what is seen or not seen:

An 80-year-old man goes to his doctor's office. The doctor says, "We need a sperm count, but we won't trouble you about that here. Take this jar home and bring back a sample tomorrow.

The man goes home. The next day he appears and presents the jar, which is as empty and clean as before. The doctor asks about this.

"I'm awful embarrassed," the man says. "First, I tried my right hand, and... nothing. Then my left hand...still nothing. Then I asked my wife. Right hand... left hand ... still nothing. She even tried with her mouth, first her teeth in, then her teeth out. We called the lady next door, you know, hands, mouth...and still nothing."

The doctor was dumbfounded and couldn't speak.

Then the man says, "Yeah, we tried everything we could think of, and we still couldn't get the jar open!"

And then there's this one:

A receptionist tells the doctor, "Oh you're going to love this patient, a real nut case. He's out there in the waiting room, and he told me he's invisible."

"Oh that is good. Well, you can just tell him I can't see him now."

☙   ☙   ☙

A much-beloved cardiologist died and the community set about creating an elaborate funeral. There were valentine hearts everywhere at the church and at the graveside, even the limousine that transported the casket was covered with hearts.

At the graveside an imposing mausoleum of pink marble stood ready to receive the casket. It was shaped like a heart. The casket rested in front of the mausoleum until the ceremonies had finished, then enormous doors swung open and the casket was wheeled in. The doors closed with a resounding thump and there were many tears among those assembled.

Except for one man, who laughed heartily.

Bystanders tried to shush him but to no avail. Someone asked him why he was being so irreverent.

"Because...," he gasped out between guffaws, "I know I'll die some day... and perhaps I'll have a fancy ceremony...and I'm a gynecologist!

A bystander nearby fainted dead away. He was the town's proctologist.

TOUCH

A man has gone to visit his doctor for a routine check-up. Upon returning home, he describes the prostate check to his wife.

"And then he put one hand on one shoulder, and the other hand on my other shoulder, and then...Oh, my God!"

In this story, the presumed sodomy of the doctor suggests the fears and vulnerabilities of the male patient. To be raped per anum becomes a symbol of the indignity of being a patient and submitting to the will and power of another man. He becomes the imaginative interpreter of sensuous imagery, allowing us to follow along with his discovery.

A blonde [or some other minority] goes to her doctor, complaining of pain.

"Where does it hurt?" asks the doctor.

"It hurts here (she touches her arm) and here (she touches her shoulder) and here [joke can be extended to any length].

"Oh, I see," says the doctor. "It's all too clear: you've broken your finger."

This somewhat macabre joke has been around a long time:

A man is waking up from surgery. "Oh doctor!"

"What's the matter?"

"I can't feel anything!"

"Now, now, don't you worry. In a case like this, it's perfectly normal."

"Oh, that's good."

"Well, you see: we removed your hands."

Hands and fingers are, of course, very important to us; we fear their loss and sometimes joke about it:

A man loses all his fingers in an accident at the sawmill. The ambulance rushes him to a hospital some distance away.

"Oh jeez," says the doctor, "but I've had pretty good luck with reattachments. Give me the fingers, and I'll see what I can do."

"Oh heck, doc. I don't have them."

"What do you mean? This is the modern age, with microsurgery, chilled tissue techniques, and on and on!"

"Well, I tried, but I just couldn't pick them up!"

And then there's this one:

"Doctor, doctor, you must help me!"

"Well, what is the matter?"

"My hands shake all the time!"

"Well, do you drink?"

"No! I spill everything!"

This joke uses imagery of both touch and sight, as well as the dual meanings of "drink."

Hearing

A woman goes to her doctor complaining of intestinal gas, which she passes at regular intervals.

"Worse yet," she complains, "They don't make any noise."

After a thorough exam the doctor says, "We can certainly help you with your gastrointestinal problem, but based on my observations over the last 15 minutes, you'll need a hearing test as well."

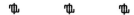

Two women are sitting on the porch at the retirement home, reminiscing about their lives.

"And did you have a good marriage?"

"Oh yes. And I missed Andy when he died. What about you?"

"It was lovely, but when Bob went, a big part of my life was gone."

"I understand. Was the sex good?"

"It was great. We had it every Sunday, listening to the bells of the church. He'd go in on the dings, and out on the dongs."

"My, that's unusual, but if it gave you pleasure...."

"Well, yes, I must say it did, but, you know, I think he'd still be with us, if it weren't for that damn Good Humor truck that went by our house."

Smell and Taste

Smell and taste are much allied senses, but in contrast to animals, these are not much used by modern, urban humans; indeed our vocabulary is weak in words to describe smells. Clearly we are affected by perfume, pheromones, smells of food, and unattractive smells, but apparently we don't like to joke about them much. I have come across few jokes using these senses. Here are two.

Why do your farts smell?

So deaf people can enjoy them too!

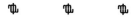

What's the difference between an oral thermometer and an anal thermometer?

The taste.

Parts Of Bodies

We turn now to jokes that employ imagery of body parts. Their energy comes from a combination of Bergsonian qualities of stiffness and mechanical nature as well as taboos concerning unhealthy bodies. Losses of body parts are, of course, psychologically traumatic, and we express some of our fear of such losses through humor that is often somewhat macabre. Some of these stories rely less on medical interventions and more on the abnormal condition that might require a visit to a hospital or doctor for treatment.

A woman meets a man on the Internet. They get in touch by phone. He has a wonderful voice; he's charming and intelligent. They exchange pictures; he's very handsome. They make a date, skipping a neutral location such as a coffee bar. Instead he's to come to her house. She spends the afternoon bathing, doing her hair, selecting her clothes, fixing her makeup. When the doorbell rings, she rushes to the door, opens it and looks out. She sees no one.

"What the…," she mutters.

"Down here," she hears, and looks down to see a very handsome man lying on the floor of her porch. He has no arms or legs.

"Oh my gosh," she manages. "You know, I mean, gosh, I mean, I just don't think this is going to work out."

He quickly replies, "I rang the doorbell, didn't I?"

In this joke, the taboo body part, the penis—erect, we suppose—is not mentioned but suggested, leaving the hearer/reader to imagine how he rang. (A similar non-mentioning of the penis is in William Carlos Williams' poem "Danse Russe," in which his naked dancing is extensively but not completely described.)

HEADS

Our culture is very head-centered. We often look at each others' faces to assess physical attractiveness and/or emotional reactions. We consider the brain to be the most important organ and believe that rational thought is the pinnacle of mental experience. Speech comes from the head and many important sense organs are located there: sight, hearing, taste, and smell. In many cultures, hanging, decapitation, and shooting a person in the head have been a means of execution. Waterboarding is head-specific. Given all the values we attach to the head, the humor about heads is especially vivid.

At a swim meet for the physically handicapped, swimmers with various problems take their places at the end of the pool, leaving one empty lane. There's a bustle in the crowd nearby, and a head (with no body whatsoever) rolls out to the edge of the pool and takes its place in the lineup.

The other contestants stare and look away quickly, carefully taking their marks for the race.

When the starter's gun goes off, all dive in and swim like crazy; even the head rolls off the edge of the pool, making a splash such as a cannon ball might make. And it sinks to the bottom of the pool.

Officials jump in and drag the head up to the surface. They push it onto the edge of the pool.

It coughs and spits out water.

Then it shouts, "Oh my gosh! What a time to get a cramp!"

Another tradition involves heads of babies.

A man is in the waiting room while his wife gives birth. When the doctor comes out, the man jumps up with joy, but then he sees a sad look on the doctor's face.

"I hate to tell you this, but your son was born without arms and legs. In fact, he has no torso either.

"What?"

"Yes, he's just a head, but he has nice brown eyes."

So the man loves his son anyway and raises him as best he can. When the boy is 18, the man takes him to the neighborhood bar for his first drink. Everyone there knows about the boy's condition and is kind and supportive. Indeed, they help pour beer down his mouth. After four drinks, however, a miracle occurs, and two legs pop out from the base of his skull.

Elated at his new legs, the boy careens across the bar, out the door, across the sidewalk, and into the street, where he is crushed by a Greyhound bus.

The men at the bar rush after him, too late. Standing in the door, the bartender wipes his eyes with his towel and says, "He should have quit while he was a head!"

There are other similar jokes, including a baby that is only an eyeball (but it's blind!), only an ear (but it's deaf!), and so on. Those jokes somewhat dramatically represent our fears that our offspring will be incomplete; they are the opposite of the ritual phrase in the birthing room, when all ten fingers have been counted: "your baby is perfect," even though other deficits, for example developmental delays, are still quite possible.

Another variation of head jokes starts with a normal (if defunct) head:

When Mr. Jones died, he was taken to a funeral home, where he was prepared for the viewing. His wife brought in his favorite blue suit, so that he could be laid out properly. On the day of the funeral, however, she arrived a few minutes early and was horrified to see him in a brown suit that she had never seen, and she was quite sure it wasn't his.

She complained loudly to the staff, "You have the wrong suit and people are parking out front even now as we speak! If you don't have him correctly dressed immediately, I'll sue your asses for 19 million dollars!"

The undertaker apologized profusely and directed an assistant to comfort Mrs. Jones. The undertaker wheeled the casket out, while Mrs. Jones and the assistant went outside to slow down the arriving crowd.

When they came into the viewing room in a few minutes, there was the late Mr. Brown at peace in his blue suit. Mrs. Brown was sure that a miracle had occurred, and the rest of the obsequies went most smoothly.

Afterwards, the assistant asked the undertaker, "How the hell did you pull that off?"

"Trade secret," he replied.

"No, really."

"It is a trade secret...but as you are an up-and-coming young man, sure to do well in this business, I will share it with you. The blue suit was put on another deceased of comparable stature, so I simply switched the heads."

PROSTHESES JOKES

At least in theory, H. Bergson would like jokes about parts of humans that are totally mechanical. Whether he would like the outrageous puns in the two following must remain an open question.

A young man is shy because his skin is entirely purple. After years of loneliness and indecision, he makes the bold move of going to a singles bar. He sits near a young woman at the bar, also very shy. Neither can say anything, but they drink enormous quantities of beer. Suddenly she emits a very large belch, her body lurching on the stool, and a glass eye pops out of her head. The young man, who has been good at sports, catches it, wipes it off on a napkin and hands it back to her.

"Say," he says, blushing, "I've been noticing you."

"Well, isn't that a coincidence," she says, "because you just happened to catch my eye!"

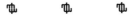

Another young man is shy because he has a prosthetic eye made of wood, but painted so expertly that no on can tell. Nonetheless, he stays home for years, finally going to a mixer, hoping to meet a young lady. He stands off to the side for most of the dance, but finally sees a young woman similarly avoiding other people, a classic wallflower. He goes over to her and notices that she has a hare-lip. His heart leaps, knowing full well her sadness and difficulty with social situations.

He says, "Say, would you like to dance?" She exclaims joyfully, "Would I, would I, would I?" [wood eye]

To which, he cries back, "Harelip, harelip, harelip!"

Because she unwittingly names his taboo secret, he feels anger that erupts in naming her defect. In this joke, both characters are scapegoats, symbols of our fears concerning physical appearance and social acceptance.

A more elaborate joke takes an unexpected turn of punishment:

A man who is embarrassed by his baldness and his wooden leg is, nonetheless, invited to a Halloween party. He doesn't have much social experience, but he finds a costume store on the Web. Fortunately he has some time, so he writes them a letter to ask their advice, given his two problems, which he carefully describes.

A few days later he received a parcel with the following note:

Dear Sir, Please find enclosed a pirate's outfit. The spotted scarf will cover your bald head, and, with your wooden leg, you will be just right as a pirate. Very truly yours, Ace Costumes.

The man thinks this is terrible because they have emphasized his wooden leg and so he writes a letter of complaint. A week goes by and he receives another parcel and a note, which says:

Dear Sir, Please find enclosed a monk's habit. The long robe will cover your wooden leg and, with your bald head, you will really look the part. Very truly yours, Ace Costumes.

Now the man is really upset since they have gone from emphasizing his wooden leg to emphasizing his bald head, so again he writes the company another nasty letter of complaint.

The next day he gets a small parcel and a note, which reads:

Dear Sir, Please find enclosed a bottle of molasses and a bag of crushed nuts. Pour the molasses over your bald head, pat on crushed nuts, then stick your wooden leg up your ass and go as a caramel apple. Very truly yours, Ace Costumes.

MALE GENITALIA

While out for a morning jog, a young man found a brand new tennis ball. He looked around for a possible owner and, finding none, shoved the ball—with some difficulty—into the pocket of his running shorts.

Soon he stopped for a red light, waiting for the WALK sign. A young woman also waiting noticed the extraordinary bulge in his shorts and lustfully asked, "Well, what's this you have here?"

"Tennis ball," he said.

"Oh dear," she said with sympathy, her eyebrows knitting in concern, "that must be very painful. I know: I had tennis elbow once."

Besides the obvious puns, we have a selective form of gigantism here, that some aspect (or all aspects) of male genitalia are enormous. The unlikely behavior of the woman suggests a male interest in sexually aggressive women.

A Cure for Headaches

After years of suffering from terrible headaches, Steve decided to see his doctor.

The doctor said, "Steve, the good news is I can cure your headaches; the bad news is that it will require castration. You have a very rare condition which causes your testicles to press on your spine, and the pressure creates one hell of a headache. The only way to relieve the pressure is to remove the testicles."

Steve was shocked and depressed, but decided he had no choice but to go under the knife. After convalescing, he decided it would be good for his morale to get some new clothes.

He entered the menswear shop and told the salesman, "I'd like a new suit."

The elderly tailor eyed him briefly and said, "Let's see...size 44 long."

Steve laughed, "That's right, how did you know?"

"Been in the business over 60 years."

Steve tried on the suit. It fit perfectly.

As Steve admired himself in the mirror, the salesman asked, "How about a new shirt?" Steve thought for a moment and then said, "Sure."

The salesman eyed Steve and said, "Let's see, 34 sleeve and 16-1/2 neck."

Steve was surprised, "That's right, how did you know?"

"Been in the business 60 years!"

Steve tried on the shirt, and it fit perfectly.

As Steve adjusted the collar in the mirror, the salesman asked, "How about some new shoes?"

Steve was on a roll and said, "Sure."

The salesman eyed Steve's feet and said, "Let's see...9-1/2E.

Steve was astonished, "That's right, how did you know?"

"Been in the business 60 years!"

Steve tried on the shoes and they fit perfectly. Steve walked comfortably around the shop and the salesman asked, "How about some new underwear?"

Steve thought for a second and said, "Sure."

The salesman stepped back, eyed Steve's waist and said, "Let's see...size 36."

Steve laughed, "Ah ha! I got you this time! I've worn size 34 since I was 18 years old."

The salesman shook his head, "You can't wear a size 34. A 34 underwear would press your testicles up against the base of your spine and give you one hell of a headache."

Here, of course, a common man is portrayed as having more knowledge (albeit whimsical) than a medical professional who performed surgery that was futile and mutilating.

Hong Kong Dong

A man goes on a trip to the Orient. He feels he has transcended the repressions of his culture and tries various exotic pleasures, including a trip to a brothel in Hong Kong.

After his return home, however, he finds that his penis is diseased and goes to his family doctor. The doctor has never seen anything like this and sends him to a urologist.

The urologist takes a look and says, "Were you traveling to the East by any chance?"

The man says he was.

"Was Hong Kong on your itinerary?"

"Yes, it was."

"Well, you've contracted a case of Hong Kong Dong."

"Is it serious?"

"I'm afraid so. The only cure is amputation."

"No!" the man exclaims and runs out of the office.

At home, he turns to his computer and after searching, finds an alternative healer nearby.

He makes an appointment and goes to that office.

"My urologist said amputation is the only cure!" he blurts out.

"Oh, that's not true at all," the healer advises.

"Oh, thank God," the man says.

"Not true at all. You can do nothing and in another week the afflicted organ will simply fall off."

This joke punishes the sexual adventurism of the man and satirizes the alternative healer as well.

FEMALE GENITALIA

In the following story we consider the archetypally perfect figure of Eve.

The Dilemma of Three Breasts

When God created woman originally, she had three breasts. God asked Eve whether she was satisfied with her body. Leaning over a pool in Eden, she looked at her chest.

"It looks very nice in every regard, but I do have one reservation."

"And what might that be, Eve?"

Concerned, she put a hand on the middle breast and said, "You know, I think two breasts would actually look better. Can you take off this middle one?

And God said, "Why yes, I think that's an excellent suggestion. Place your two hands below your middle breast."

She did so.

He waved his hand and the middle breast fell away into her hands, and the result was good, very good.

And the woman, looking at the breast in her hand, said, "What can be done with this useless boob?"

"Give it to me," God said.

And from it, He created man.

And women have wondered ever since whether that was good.

I've read or heard several versions of this, and there are several reasons for its popularity. There's the parody of the well known Biblical account, there's the suggestion that God is the ultimate doctor, there's the pun on "boob," (revealing men as idiots) and, of course, the feminist reversal of God creating woman from a man's rib. There's also an affirmation of the attractiveness, even perfection of women's au pair mammaries, also celebrated in the following riddle:

Q. Why is a woman's breast like a martini?

A. Because one is too little, but three are too many.

Double mammaries are not, of course, the only possibility. Statues of the Ephesian Diana, a symbol of fertility, have many, many breasts in several rows across her torso.

Other jokes about female anatomy and appearance are in SHAPE SHIFTING below, and scattered throughout this book.

ANUS, RECTUM, BUTTOCKS

There are many jokes about our fundaments, often including some version of punishment and/or degradation, as in the Easter lily joke.

In the following joke, the pain is self-inflicted.

At a leather bar, Larry sees a cute young man and is smitten with love at first sight. He asks around and learns—to his delight—that the man is a proctologist. Larry is much too shy to approach the man at the bar, so he makes an appointment at the doctor's office.

"What can I do for you?" the doctor asks.

"I have pain in my rectum," says Larry.

"O.K., let's have a look."

Larry pulls of his clothes and jumps up on the examining table.

"Good heavens," the doctor says, taking a close look, "you have a rose protruding from your anus, and there appear to be thorns on the stem. Gracious, there's even a little blood!"

Beside himself with joy, Larry cries out, "Read the card! Read the card!"

There's another joke hinging on a strange pun; I've heard several versions of this.

A woman goes to her doctor, distraught that she is unlucky in love. He counsels her, hoping that talk will be sufficient, but she insists on a full physical exam. He finds nothing out of the ordinary but suddenly has an inspiration.

"Crawl on all fours," he says, and she does so.

"Ah, just as I thought," says he.

"Is it serious?" says she.

"I'm afraid so: it's the Zachary syndrome."

"The what?"

"The Zachary syndrome: your face looks ex-zachary [exactly] like your butt."

This is assuredly not the most subtle of stories, and there are both male and female versions; either way, there's a taboo against our nether portions that is broken by equating them with our most social area, our face. Other variations include, "He was the south end of a north-bound horse." The joke criticizes a similarity (even an equation!) of face and sexual areas, perhaps a reference to taboos in this culture against sexual practices such as fellatio, cunnilingus, anilingus and anal intercourse; these taboos may be nominal, if Kinsey, Masters and Johnson, or some women's magazines are to be credited. Even the suggestion of similarity between the two ends of the body strongly breaks taboo in our head-focused culture. The physician's demand that she crawl on all fours suggests his sexual dominance while he reduces her to animal status. Thus he is also satirized in making his bizarre request.

An ingenious (if somewhat shaggy) joke using an actual horse goes like this; oddly enough it's a cousin to the cross-eyed dog we encountered earlier:

A man has always wanted a race horse—something his wife as steadfastly denied him. In his middle years, having accumulated enough money to do so, he sneaks off to an auction and buys a beautiful chestnut Arabian—a real beauty of a horse. With great pride, he brings the horse back to his estate and calls his wife to admire it.

She takes one look and says, "You fool, you've been cheated; this horse is worthless: he's cross-eyed."

"No," says the man. "Impossible!"

"See for yourself," says his wife. He goes to the front of the horse and sees, sure enough that the horse is cross-eyed. He throws his hat on the ground and jumps up and down on it. Then he calls the seller and demands his money back.

The seller says, "Caveat emptor, which is Latin for let the buyer beware. In other words: tough luck and/or you lose."

The man calls a veterinarian, who travels out to the estate. After examining the horse he confirms that the horse is in fact cross-eyed, but the good news is that he can repair the damage.

"Go ahead," says the man.

"OK, you stand in front while I operate."

The man stands in front while the vet reaches into his black bag and pulls out a chrome pipe. He raises the horse's tail and twists the pipe into the anus.

"Ready?" he calls.

"Ready!"

The vet blows on the pipe, and the man standing in front is delighted to see that the horse's eyes straighten out.

"Wow, that's great. Thank you!"

"You're very welcome and that'll be $1,000 for today."

"What? For five minutes' work?"

"Are the eyes straight, or are they not?"

The man grudgingly pays then goes to get his wife so that she can see that the horse is now perfect.

She comes out, takes a look, and pronounces the horse cross-eyed.

The man looks, and sees that she's right. He starts to call the vet but remembers the expensive fee for service.

Accordingly, he goes to his shop and finds a similar pipe. He orders his wife to the front of the horse. He inserts the pipe and blows on it.

She calls back that nothing has improved.

She also yells, "You're not doing it right!"

She orders him to the front of the horse.

She marches to the back of the horse, and removes the pipe from the horse. She turns it around and re-inserts it.

"Hey, why are you doing that?" the husband calls.

"Well," she calls back, "I certainly wasn't going to put my mouth where yours was!"

A thoroughly silly and unlikely joke, this text manages to combine criticism of a greedy veterinarian and a hectoring female, as well as the mechanical cure for crossed eyes through air pressure, with, of course, an exaggerated sense of sanitation (reminiscent of many male-female conflicts in households) on the part of the wife, which is punished by whatever the horse has in its rectum. For better or worse, the senses of sight, touch, smell, and perhaps taste are all evoked.

There are many jokes about excrement and flatulence, let's close this section with two, reminiscent of grade-school humor.

Q. Why is your ass groove vertical and not horizontal?

A. So that your cheeks won't vibrate when you slide down a banister.

Q. Why are your turds tapered?

A. So your asshole won't slam shut.

Multiple Parts

One day when Hal and Jim were out cutting wood, Jim cut his arm off. Accustomed to accidents in the woods, Hal calmly wrapped the arm in a plastic tarp and brought Jim to the nearest hospital.

"Today is your lucky day," said the ER doctor. "We just happen to have a great reattachment surgeon on staff. Come back in six hours."

Hal comes back to see how Jim is doing. The surgeon says, "Your buddy did great. In fact, he's down at the bar, and, if I'm not mistaken, he'll be playing darts with the arm I put back on." Hal goes to the bar and finds Jim playing darts.

The next month, Hal and Jim are out cutting wood, when Jim cuts off a leg. Hal wraps the limb in a plastic tarp and takes Jim to the same hospital. The same surgeon says, "Well, legs are a little harder, but if you come back in eight hours, you'll be pleasantly surprised." Hal does so and learns that Jim is in the park kicking a soccer ball.

The next month, Hal and Jim are out cutting wood, and Jim cuts off his head. Hal wraps the head in a plastic tarp and takes Jim to the same hospital. The same surgeon says, "Heads are very difficult. Come back in 10 hours.

Hal comes back in ten hours, and the surgeon says, "I'm so sorry, but your friend is dead."

"Oh no," cries Hal, "I thought you could do just about anything!"

"Oh, I can, for sure. In fact, I reattached the head perfectly, but unfortunately it had already suffocated in the tarp you used."

This bizarre joke has resonances with Adam and Eve, the Tower of Babel, Prometheus, and Frankenstein ("the Modern Prometheus," in Mary Shelley's subtitle), stories that present the ambitions of humans to control the world and their inevitable failures. Hal (and many of us) believe that modern medicine can do almost anything; as a result, we are sometimes disappointed, shamed, and/or devastated when medicine cannot repair our mortal bodies.

SHAPE SHIFTING: CHANGES IN BODY IMAGE THROUGH PLASTIC SURGERY

There's a long tradition of shape-shifting in folktales, sometimes through acts of the supernatural, sometimes through magic, sometimes through fantasy. In modern times, however, plastic surgery is the common means to physically change a person's looks. Given our intense concern about aging, jokes about plastic surgery are common, dramatic, and even outrageous. At this writing, various TV shows feature plastic surgery: we see images of the body before and after, even with commentary during the surgery. Evidently there are sufficient audiences to keep these shows on the air. There are also many jokes readily available, such as the following.

The Knob

A woman has had several face-lifts. Finally her surgeon tells her there is nothing more he can do for her: he's trimmed, tucked, and lifted all he can.

She protests and badgers him until he refers her to another—and less reputable—surgeon who has an experimental technique called "The Knob."

At a consultation with him, she learns that he'll install a knob on the top of her head; it will be cleverly concealed in her hair. Whenever she needs a tightening up of her face, she'll need merely to reach up and turn the knob. Delighted, she consents to the operation.

And another year goes by, during which she uses the knob many times.

One day she awakes to find large bags under her eyes. Alarmed, she calls the doctor's office; the nurse advises her to come right over. She takes a cab. Soon she's in an examining room.

"Oh, dear," says the doctor. "I'm afraid I must tell you that those bags are actually your breasts."

"Oh my," says she, "and I guess that would explain the goatee."

While this joke is cheerfully absurd in its exaggeration, women have had, in my lifetime, teeth removed to create hollow cheeks, the twelfth rib removed for a narrower waist, and the little toes removed for a smaller foot that can wear shoes with pointed toes, as well as facelifts, Botox injections, tattoos, and liposuction—all quite common today, and not just for women. The joke parodies the vanity of the woman and the greed of the second surgeon, who will do work well beyond standards of care. The imagery of the knob and its hoisting ability are wildly exaggerated. That she is complicit in working the mechanical knob is a further source of our scornful laughter. To have her face demeaned by a man-like beard is funny too, since she wanted to be more attractive as a woman; the "goatee" is, of course, her pubic hair—a subject usually not mentioned in this culture, another taboo. We pay tribute to the sexual maturity of a woman by not mentioning this feature, and other hair (on legs, armpits, chins, and cheeks) is typically removed (or lessened, in the case of eyebrows) to suggest that she is neotonous, that is, like a young woman just coming into her earliest and most attractive sexual maturity.

There's also a male version of pride seeking a solution through plastic surgery.

Morton, at 105 years of age, decides he really should do something about the many wrinkles in his skin. When he reads of a bold new technique, he is interested: the surgeon hoists the anesthetized patient up to the ceiling, from which he dangles, attached only by his scalp. Gravity pulls his body down, and all loose skin is pulled upwards, so that the surgeon can cut it off and close up neatly.

Morton has the operation. Upon leaving the hospital, he meets someone who looks vaguely familiar; this man speaks to him hesitantly.

"Morton, is that you?"

"Yes."

"Well, I can barely recognize you."

"I just had extensive plastic surgery...and who are you?"

"I'm Frank, but I'm not surprised you don't recognize me. I had plastic surgery also. Say, I don't remember that you had a dimple on your chin."

"I didn't. That's my navel."

"Ha ha ha, but I can go you one better. Get a look at what I'm wearing for a tie!"

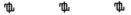

God Makes a Mistake

A middle-aged woman suffers a heart attack; an ambulance takes her to the nearest Emergency Room. ER doctors send her for cardiac surgery during which she has a near-death experience, going through the tunnel, seeing people in white robes and, finally, God himself on a golden throne.

She falls on her knees, clasps her hands, looks up, and whispers, "Lord, is this really my time to die?"

He replies in a deep, rumbling voice, "My dear child, no—it is not. I grant you another 30 years, six months, 27 days, and change."

The surgery is a success and, while recovering, she decides to make the best of her remaining years. Accordingly, she stays in the hospital for a face-lift, a boob job, a tummy tuck, an ass lift, and liposuction. She has her hairdresser come to the hospital to tint her hair a new color.

Finally, she leaves the hospital. Walking across the street she is hit by another ambulance (or maybe the same one?) and killed on the spot.

Arriving before God, she says, "Hey! Whatever happened to the 30 years plus you promised me!"

God replies, "Oh, for Heavens' sake." He slaps His brow. "I didn't recognize you!"

In Summary

Our bodies allow us to move and to manipulate objects; they allow us to perceive the world; they allow us to enjoy sports, love-making, and all sensuous pleasures. They also have limitations, even though our desires and imaginations often yearn for more strength, more durability, and more mobility. When we are injured or sick, we lose some of our physical capacities. If we are seriously injured or very sick, we must deal with profound physical losses and consider the possibility of the complete loss of our bodies, which is to say death.

Humor about body parts and processes is one of our coping mechanisms, a way of maintaining imaginative health. By our use of language and corporeal imagery, we break the taboos that limit sensible and sensitive discussion of bodily realities. In sharing such jokes, we redefine our emotions—fears in particular—about our bodies, and we create comic communities that help us see that others share our own personal nervousness about bodies, so that we may see ourselves as normal. We also affirm that interest in bodies' healthy appearance is important and even necessary to the continuance of the race. We affirm, as well, the power and freedom of the imagination to deal with these difficult issues. Furthermore, we situate ourselves closer to a center of normality by imaginatively extending the far borders of abnormality in extreme, even outrageous humor about bodies and body parts. Jokes about the body not only draw our attention to our bodies, but also allow us to change our emotional evaluations of them. And, when sickness and healing are involved, we have the possibilities of new wisdom about how we live in our bodies.

Chapter Seven

Humour Characters and Their Stories

DOCTOR VISIT: PATIENT ON A SHORT LEASH

ONE VISIT TO my doctor ended with these words: "Well, Howard, I'm going to keep you on a short leash for this one. How about you come back in two weeks?" Although I didn't really want to come back that soon, I enjoyed his implied metaphor that I was a dog that might run away, while he was the master who made choices concerning leash length. Through this joke, he made fun of himself as a dog handler and of our enforced relationship that implied his power and my obedience. The patient's role sometimes makes me feel like an animal, so I'm always thankful for a doctor or nurse or technician who can make a gentle joke when I'm a patient, thus assuring me that I'm still a human. Such a person entertains me and suggests that I still belong to the world of the well, even while I'm in the world of the sick—temporarily, I hope.

WHY HUMOUR CHARACTERS ARE HUMOROUS

When I was a young professor of literature, I emphasized plot as the first element of fiction. After all, Aristotle's *Poetics* said the plot was the soul of tragedy and, by extension, of all narratives. But as semesters rolled by, I came to believe that looking at characters was a better starting point, since the figures of plays, poems, and stories are images of people, and we, as readers, are also people who relate to them. I noticed that students, especially women, tended to talk about characters first and story second, and their insights into what characters desired or feared were usually crucial to motivation. And motivation—as Aristotle also pointed out—was a driver for plot. Furthermore, characters' reactions to events guide our reactions as we read a text or see a play or a movie.

We'll turn to stories in a moment, but first let's look at the curious creatures that make them all possible, that enliven them and draw us into their worlds. Without characters there can be no story. Furthermore, whether the humor is in the Emergency

Room or by the water cooler, it's people who make the jokes, and the stories in the jokes always involve people as characters, even if the characters appear as animals.

We speak of characters because, obviously, they have character, or *characteristics* that stand out, especially in comic literature. There can be no subtle Gargantua, no bland Falstaff, no quiet Lucille Ball. In Chapter One we briefly discussed humour characters, noting that their personality was based on predominance of one of the four humours: blood, phlegm, yellow bile, or black bile. (We saw a chart of the humours in Figure 3.1 in Chapter Three.) A strong predominance of one humour in a person challenged social order, and comedy would either correct the balance in that person or exile him/her as a scapegoat. Let's review the four humours and their uses in jokes people tell about medical topics. In the discussion that follows, I draw heavily on John W. Draper's monograph *The Humors & Shakespeare's Characters*.[1] While Draper and others commonly use the "humor" spelling, I will use "humour" to indicate the body fluids that influence character, but "humor" to indicate something funny. For each humour, I'll describe a cartoon from *The New Yorker Book of Doctor Cartoons* that illustrates the concept.[2]

BLOOD: SEX, EXTROVERSION, SEX, HEROISM, AND MORE SEX

Peter Arno's cartoon shows four men appreciatively examinng the belly of an attractive woman who smiles, her arms upraised. Off to the side, a nurse tells another (apparently younger) nurse: "Humph! You'd think it was the first appendectomy they ever saw" (p. 6).

In the ancient psychology of humours, blood was associated with the element air, the qualities of hot and wet, and a temperament called "sanguine," which meant vital and active, for example a person of good spirits and sexual energy. The parallel season is spring; a time of reawakening, vitality, and breeding. For Shakespeare, this was the best humour to predominate in a person, and his heroes and lovers are sanguine types, including, of course, the lovesick Romeo. Fielding's Tom Jones is another sanguine character, a man always ready for sex. When we are sick or injured, however, we typically feel most un-sanguine and yearn for our return to the world of the well and its vitality.

In popular culture, we often project our fears upon doctors and nurses, whom we imagine as ridiculously sanguine: enjoying life, wealth, health, and sex willy-nilly, while sick people are deprived, left out, even exiled. Sometimes there is also jealousy of doctors' prestige, wealth, and power, all targets for satire, as in the following joke:

> At a cocktail party an alluring blonde comes up to Dr. Flynn and greets him warmly.

"Who was that?" Dr. Flynn's wife asks accusingly.

"Why, that's my mistress," Dr. Flynn states.

"What? I'm calling a lawyer in the morning!" she screams at him.

"OK, but before you do, think about the house you enjoy, the club, the private school for our kids, the job you don't have to have, the cars, the vacations, and so on."

A gorgeous brunette walks by.

"Who's that?" Mrs. Flynn asks.

"Oh, that's Dr. Stevens' mistress."

Says the wife, "Ours is prettier."

Here the doctor is sanguine, enjoying sex beyond social norms: he's an adulterer. And predictably, his wife castigates him. By the end of the joke, however, she is as corrupt as he is, because she benefits economically and socially by his position, and we laugh at both of them. Furthermore, Dr. Stevens also has a mistress, and who knows how many other doctors do as well? So we laugh at such libidinous doctors as a whole class of corrupt characters.

It's not always sanguine doctors who are the humorous target. We saw this one-liner earlier: Did you hear about the nurse who could make the patient without disturbing the bed?

Sometimes it's a patient who is sanguine beyond normality:

A woman goes to her doctor to complain that she is often tired in the morning. After a series of diagnostic tests, the doctor is not finding anything significant. Striking out into behavioral areas, he asks her how often she has intercourse.

"Oh that? Gosh, it's every Monday, Wednesday, and Saturday night."

"Aha!" says the doctor, "now we're getting somewhere. I'd advise you to cut out Wednesday and see how your energy perks up."

"I follow your reasoning, doctor, but I really can't do that," says she. "That's the only night I'm home with my husband."

The medical encounter often suggests the kind of intimacy in body and mind that we associate with sexual closeness. One nervous rejection of this is through humor, as in the following joke:

A lady goes to the dentist, who finds a brown spot on one of her teeth.

"I'm going to have to drill this out," he says.

"Damn," she says, "I'd rather have a child."

"Oh well, in that case," says the dentist, "let me adjust the chair."

Whether we are making jokes about sex or watching *Romeo and Juliet*, we care a lot about sexual attractiveness of humans and how they become loving couples. Humor is one way of acknowledging such desires and, at the same time, our fears about loss of vitality and power if we become sick.

Yellow Bile: Anger, High Energy, Obsession, Mania

Donald Reilly's cartoon shows an angry physician behind his desk. While a patient leaves in the background, a nurse says, "Doctor, you *must* stop addressing your Medicare patients as Comrade" (p. 4).

According to humour theory, yellow bile was associated with fire (hot, dry) and a personality that is angry or choleric ("choler" is another word for bile). The parallel season is summer, a time of intense heat and maximal growth of crops. Shakespeare loved these characters for their high energy and strong resolve, all of which made for good drama. Othello, Iago, and Henry V are among the choleric male leads. The choleric females often had less to do on stage, but they typically defied their parents (the shrew Kate, Juliet, and Lear's three daughters, Goneril, Regan, and even Cordelia).

The choleric figure is angry, a mad person, perhaps someone possessed with an obsession or a mania. In the medical world, it is often the intensity of doctors (surgeons in particular) that becomes a target for satire. One real-life example I recall from my Emergency Room was a doctor who dialed out on two telephones to another doctor's office then stood between them, holding both handpieces to his ears and crowing, "Now I've got both of his phones tied up!"

Another feature of cholerics is that they are good, even aggressive talkers. Comedians and jokers in general enjoy bending or breaking taboos, sometimes just for the fun of it, but also sometimes in anger to subvert the prudishness or oppression of society or, through satire, to correct unhealthy imbalances of society.

Some choleric humor attacks doctors, whom we sometimes blame for our medical dilemmas. We satirize doctors as controllers (playing God) and persons who boss us around. Our revenge is through satiric humor, for example portraying doctors as manipulative:

A man has been feeling down in the dumps for some time. Finally he goes to the doctor for a complete physical.

"Well," says the doctor, "I'm afraid the news I have for you is not good."

"Oh, no," says the man. "But give it to me straight."

"OK...the fact is you are dying."

"Good Lord! How much time do I have?"

"Ten," says the doctor.

"Ten? Ten what? Years? Months? Weeks?"

"Nine."

Sometimes the patient attacks the doctor:

A doctor tells his patient, "I'm sorry to trouble you, Mr. Jones, but we're going to need a urine sample, a stool sample, and a semen sample."

"Oh, that's OK, doc. Here, take my underpants."

MELANCHOLY: THE BLUES, SADNESS, FEAR, DEPRESSION

Robert Kraus's cartoon shows a doctor listening to the chest of a sad clown, while three circus people just outside wait hopefully. The doctor says, "Good heavens, man, your heart is breaking!" (p. 36).

The word "melancholy" is made up of the Greek roots *melan* ("black") and *choly* ("choler" or "bile"). In the modern usage, melancholy means sadness, but in earlier times it included depression and fearfulness as well (all lengthily explored in Robert Burton's *Anatomy of Melancholy*, 1621). The traditional qualities for this humour were dry and cold, and the element was earth, the heaviest of the four elements. Jokes in this area emphasize the *stuff*—often inflexible—of our bodies, as we saw in Chapter Six. Shakespeare created some great twisted melancholics, including Richard III (a hunchback), the bastard Edmund, the senile King Lear, and even the later Romeo. The season of the year is fall, when greenery shrivels and pathetically dies.

Melancholics are worriers, gloom-mongers, sad sacks. As comic characters, they express the doubts and fears we often carry without recognizing or expressing them. In Aristotelian terms, they need a healthy catharsis (a word related to "cathartic," a modern agent for emptying the bowels). Here's a real-life character I remember from my college days: A pre-med student was recognized by his peers to be a melancholic: he always worried and complained. One evening, his friends teased him, imagining him as a practicing physician seeing a patient. They mimicked what he'd say: "Oh my God! That looks terrible. I've never seen anything worse! Lady, you're going to die!"

By naming and exaggerating some of our deepest fears, melancholic humor tells us that our fears are not specific to us but generic through the human race. Further, they raise our fears to consciousness and help to dispel them—at least for the moment. Moviegoers will remember Woody Allen's character obsessing over a possible brain tumor in "Hannah and Her Sisters" (1986), and many were thrilled to see someone who was more of a hypochondriac than they.

I have not encountered jokes in popular culture that are obviously melancholic. I suppose the characters are uninteresting for purposes of humor, and true melancholy, such as the illness of depression, is not currently considered a joking matter in this eager-beaver, get-up-and-go society.

PHLEGM: LAZY, INERT, THE COUCH-POTATO

William Steig's cartoon portrays a nurse dragging in a limp man, while the doctor, robust and hale, booms, "Well, what seems to be the trouble, Mr. Sims?" (p. 1).

Phlegm (or mucus or snot) is surely the unloveliest humour, all cold and wet. Its element is water, and its temperament is phlegmatic or, worse, lazy. The phlegmatic person is not only lazy, but also cowardly and/or stupid. He (or she) is passive, almost inert. Such a person doesn't have much dramatic potential, and Shakespeare used them sparingly, often as women or children (unformed folks who might evolve to be dominated by another humour as they matured). Still, they make fine satiric targets, such as Falstaff, the greedy and conniving but also lazy and corpulent guzzler and gourmand. The symbolic season is winter, a time of chill, cold, and death. Phlegmatic humor is about the passivity and weakness we feel as patients, when we suffer through a time of enforced weakness and waiting. Being phlegmatic may, however, have some positive values: a nasty cold that holds us down for several days may be a time to reflect on what our lives mean, how we will act, and how we will allot our time and energy once we are well.

Phlegm can be the opposite of sanguine: a true phlegmatic is uninvolved in life, a figure to be satirized:

> A businessman was walking down the street when he was accosted by a particularly dirty and shabby-looking homeless man who asked him for a couple of dollars for a meal.
>
> The businessman took out his wallet, extracted a ten-dollar bill, extended it to the homeless man and asked, "If I give you this money, will you buy some booze with it and get drunk?"
>
> "No," said the poor fellow. "I had to stop drinking years ago."
>
> "I bet you'll gamble it away instead of buying food."
>
> "No, I don't gamble," the homeless man stated. "I need everything I can get just to stay alive."
>
> "Then I bet you spend this on greens fees at the golf course down the road."
>
> "No sir! I haven't played golf in over 20 years."
>
> "Sure! You'll spend it on a woman in the red light district, then."
>
> "Are you NUTS? And get some horrible disease for a lousy 10 bucks?"
>
> The businessman pondered a minute and put the bill back in his wallet as he stated, "I'm not going to give you any money. I'm going to take you home for a terrific home-cooked meal prepared by my wife."
>
> The homeless man was astounded. "But won't your wife be upset with you for bringing someone as filthy and smelly as me into your home?"

"Probably," replied the businessman. "But I want her to see what a man looks like after he gives up booze, gambling, golf, and sex."

Here a sanguine person satirizes a person uninvolved in life's passions and the joke makes the phlegmatic character a scapegoat on the margins of a society—which is actually shown to be corrupt.

A Phlegmatic Variation: Stupidity Jokes

Earlier we saw the joke about a man who wanted the medical term for laziness so he could relay it to his wife, but I have found few jokes about laziness. Jokers seem to prefer the sanguine and choleric humours, which provide lively characters for stories. Another phlegmatic quality, stupidity, is, however, a juicy target for satire. Jokes about dumb people from certain regions, countries, or ethnicities have been around for a while; in the 1970s, it was a series of Polish jokes. In Ohio, it's Kentucky jokes. In Canada it's Newfie jokes, and so on. The maligned group symbolizes aspects of humans in general (even including ourselves) that are stupid, especially in the face of something complex or overwhelming, such as a medical dilemma. Another subgroup, much satirized in the 1990s were Rednecks, as in the following two jokes. (The language play here attempts a satiric approximation of an uneducated, rural dialect.)

A mountain woman went to the doctor and was told to go home and come back in a couple of days with a specimen.

When she got home, she asked her husband, "Now just what do you reckon a specimen might be?"

"Well damnit, woman, how the hell would I know? You just go over yonder and ask Agnes. She wuz a nurse oncet upon a time."

So the woman leaves.

Half an hour she's back, but her clothes are all torn and she has cuts and bruises just about everywhere.

"Tarnation, woman! What the devil happened over yonder?"

"I don't rightly know, she replied. "I asked Agnes what she reckoned a specimen might be."

"Well, of course...that's why you went, ain't it?"

"You betcha, but she went and told me to go piss in a bottle. Can you believe it? So I told her she could just go shit in her hat, and then all hell broke loose."

Stupidity joke number two:

In a neighboring cabin, up there in the hills, a very pregnant woman cries out to her husband, "Clem, saddle up the mule and fetch the doc. My time is well nigh here!"

Clem saddles up the mule and rides down the mountain to find the doctor.

Says the doctor. "Are you sure? I don't want to go all the way up there for nothing."

Clem says, "Heck no, I'm not sure. I just don't know about these things. But the way she was yelling and hollering and carrying on sure looked like the real thing."

When they return to the cabin, it's growing dark. The doc examines the woman as best he can in the dim light and agrees the birth is imminent, but he also complains about the dim lighting.

"Say now, Clem, I'm going to need more light here. You hold that lantern closer."

Soon a baby arrives, and the doctor catches it and helps it breathe.

"Hold that lantern close," he says, "I gotta see to the afterbirth. But...oh my gosh...I think there's yet another baby in there!"

Sure enough, he delivers a second baby. Clem, in his excitement becomes inattentive about the lantern, and the doctor urges him one more time, "Hold that lantern close!" and once more, discovers another baby waiting to be born.

As the third baby emerges, Clem says, "Three babies—I'll be hornswoggled. Say, doc, how could that ever be? Do you think it's the lantern that's drawing them?"

One of the most popular phlegmatic characters in the past dozen years has been the blonde, possibly an offshoot of "dumb blondes" from the movies. Here's a joke that combines blonde stupidity (or naïve ignorance) with city-slicker lack of rural experience.

Jill, a big-city girl, works as a stewardess. On one of her flights she meets a Texas rancher. They fall in love and marry. At home on the ranch, Jill finds she has a lot to learn.

One day her husband has to travel to pick up some machinery. He sits Jill down and asks her if she can take care of one chore while he's gone. She smiles and agrees.

"OK, it's this. The artificial insemination man is coming, probably about noon, to impregnate our prize Holstein cow. Now, I already drove a big shiny spike into the 2x4 over her stall in the barn. Do you follow me so far?"

Jill smiles and nods.

"OK, good. So when the man arrives, I want you to take him over to the barn and show him where the cow is located. OK?

Jill smiles and nods. Her husband departs, and she watches the road to her ranch house.

Sure enough, about 12:00 the man arrives. She greets him and takes him to the barn and to the stall.

"What's that big nail doing up there?" asks the man.

Jill frowns and puts her finger to her cheek.

"Well, gosh, I guess that must be for you to hang your trousers while you do the insemination!"

Stupidity is the subject of the Darwin Awards, a real-life selection of bizarre stories published on the Web and in book form; see Wendy Northcutt, *The Darwin Awards 4: Intelligent Design*.[3] This book contains over 100 real life misadventures, most published in newspapers. The sarcastic concept of the awards is this: the people who have killed themselves through stupidity have done the human race a darwinian favor by eliminating their genes from reproduction. In her opening pages, Northcutt gives the example of a terrorist who mailed a letter bomb with not enough postage; when it returned to him, he opened it, thus killing himself. The mood of these bizarre accounts is strange, since these people are not clowns who remain undamaged; indeed they are real people who have died. Should we laugh? By norms of social decency, we should not. Do we laugh? Yes, or at least often. Why? Our laughter expresses our recognition of the absurdity in the world, our feelings of superiority over the victims described, and our gratitude that we have so far escaped with our lives. Our laughter is self-congratulatory in the sense that—although we have also done many stupid things—we have not done things as stupid as smoking in an ammunition warehouse (p. 197). A careful eight-page Story Index lists many of the ways humans can stupidly kill themselves, although I looked in vain for "doctor," "nurse," "hospital," and "medicine." For the latest, see www.darwinawards.com.

Our review of humour characters completed, we can turn to some other traditional characters.

ALMOST HUMAN: ANIMALS

The representation of humans in animal form has some taboo aspects, because Westerners, among others, feel there is an important distinction between humans and animals. After all, we congratulate ourselves that we have transcended any animality by virtue of our higher faculties, higher morals, language, reasoning, gentility, civilization, politesse, and so on. Animal characters are useful in stories, however, because we can pretend that they have more primal emotions, the kind we humans have presumably learned to control. Animal characters go well back into human history, serving in all sorts of folk tales, myths, and fables, of which Aesop's are perhaps the best known, at least in the West.

Humor involving animals (like the Pope jokes we saw in Chapter Five) typically emphasizes and celebrates our animal bases, showing our desires writ large and exhibiting a general disregard for social repressions. We also enjoy the hilarity of animals speaking, as if they could converse with us at our level (or we with them at their level). We even enjoy the spectacle of them as dogs, parrots, horses, etc., participating in our affairs. Animals can serve the fantasy dimension of stories very well through visual imagery of them in human roles, with their exaggerated behaviors and/or desires.

Sometimes the animal represents choleric behavior that needs to be repressed.

The Foul-Mouthed Parrot

A man, recently widowed, was lonely. On his way to work he walked by a pet store. Each morning and evening, he looked in the window, thinking that perhaps a pet might solace his lonely hours at home. None of the animals seemed to have the right quality, until one day a parrot with huge, colorful feathers appeared. Not only was this new addition prominently displayed, there was also a large sign which read "FOR SALE * CHEAP."

The man went in, discussed the bird with the shopkeeper, purchased it, and took it home.

He put the bird on a stand in his dining room and said, "Polly wants a cracker?"

The parrot replied with a burst of profanity, the like of which the man had never heard. Indeed any efforts he made for conversation were similarly greeted. The man called the store own and complained. The store owner allowed that the parrot had been owned by sailors but insisted that a deal was a deal.

Distraught, the man became increasing angry and spoke harshly to the parrot, finally threatening him with punishment. The parrot, however, persisted in its unrestrained behavior.

In a rage, the man grabbed the parrot from his stand and hustled it down the basement stairs. He jerked open the door to a large freezer and flung the parrot in. He slammed the door shut and stalked upstairs, turning off the light. He poured himself a drink and sat down to mull over the situation. After a while his anger calmed, and he began to feel guilt over what he had done. He became concerned about the parrot in the freezer and headed back to the basement. He ran down the stairs, pulled open the door and hauled out the poor parrot. The parrot was breathing shallowly and shivering violently.

Then, in hesitating groups of words—which appeared as little white puffs in the humid, basement air—it gasped out, "I'm sorry! I'm sorry! I'll talk nice! Give me a second chance!"

To which the man replied, "OK, OK, but you know what's in store if you swear again."

"I do! I do! But tell me…"

"Yes?"

"Whatever did the turkey do?"

The formerly choleric parrot has been corrected to a social normalcy by the cold and by the image of the frozen (phlegmatic) turkey. The parrot (apparently) reasons that the supermarket-dressed turkey must have behaved even worse. The man, who was temporarily choleric in throwing the parrot into the freezer, becomes more sanguine and considerate to the parrot. By the end of the joke, it appears that both have mellowed back toward more normal behavior. That the parrot should change from total profanity to reasoned speech is, of course, absurd. The imagery of the freezer (like a casket) and a basement (like in a Poe short story) give a gothic, repressive feel to the joke.

And now for two animal characters dealing with issues of sanguine (erotic) behavior:

In the Veterinarian's Waiting Room

A little Terrier and a Great Dane were sitting in the veterinarian's waiting room. Finished with their magazines, they turned to small talk about the weather, politics, the economy, and a new dog food. When these topics sputtered to a halt, the Great Dane asked the terrier, "So, why are you here?"

"Well, I'm afraid it's a rather sad story," he replied. "Last week I went on a walk with my mistress in the park, where she saw a friend of hers. Of course I had already noticed the little white Poodle this friend had on a leash. And what a dish! All fluffy and frisky, with a little bow on the top of her head. And the smell! Fantastic! The ladies drew near and talked, but I couldn't help myself. I leaped on top of the little poodle and gave it to her right there in the park BAM BAM BAM!"

"Oh my," said the Great Dane, "Good for you!"

"Well, the ladies went ballistic and jerked us apart by our leashes, screaming 'Bad dog! Bad, bad dog!'"

"Yes," said the Great Dane. "I can well imagine."

"But I did get in! And it was great. That was my first time and, I fear, my last. The sad truth is that I'm here to be neutered."

"Oh, that is very sad indeed," said the Great Dane.

There was a melancholic pause.

"And...and why are you here?" asked the Terrier.

"Well," said the Great Dane, "last week I was walking down the hall in my mistress' apartment and I heard water running in the bathroom. I looked in the door and saw that she was drawing a bath. In fact, she was entirely naked and bending over the tub to test the water. Well, the sight was ravishing and the smell was just fabulous, so I leaped on her right there and gave it to her whole-heartedly BAM BAM BAM." He clapped his forepaws together.

"Oh my God," whispered the Terrier. "Whatever are they going to do to you?"

"I'm here to have my nails clipped."

The dynamics here are neither difficult nor subtle. The "ladies" are styled as aversive to sex publicly, but in their own homes (if one woman may stand for both or all), they are ready and eager for sex, even interspecies activity, as willing and sub-missive partners. The dogs are parallels to humans in their speech and conventional behavior in a waiting room. As stand-ins for humans, they represent wish-fulfillment to act on a sexual urge impulsively and successfully, well beyond social taboos. The Terrier is a phlegmatic sort—unformed, young, inexperienced, who is to be rendered even more phlegmatic by castration, because he broke the ladies' rules of public behavior. The Great Dane is a sanguine figure, sexy, strong, aggressive, and he is rewarded for his sexual prowess by, it appears, future opportunities, once his nails are taken care of.

And, as in many good, jokes, we fill in the details. The women are delicately styled as "mistresses," a term that gains some ambiguity as the joke finishes. A fur-ther ambiguity is that their characters have two sides. First is the proper, somewhat phlegmatic persona that society encourages but, second, is the hidden, sanguine per-sona. The second, private persona (like the Pope's third condition of "big tits!") celebrates sexual activity and pleasure. The values of the joke underline (and/or hope for) women's hidden or covert sexual adventurism.

Two women are sitting on a bench smoking cigarettes. Regrettably, a light rain is falling. One woman complains, "Damn, my cigarette keeps going out in this stupid rain." The other replies, "I'm not having that problem, because I put a condom over my cigarette."

"Oh, how clever," the first replies, perhaps ironically.

Thinking it all over later, however, she feels the idea has some merit and, accordingly, goes to the drugstore. She speaks to the pharmacist, who evinces much surprise when she inquires about a condom that would be suitable for a Camel.

STORIES

Stories give us a linear set of events that happen as characters move through time. The jokes we're discussing are short, short stories, a few lines long or maybe a page, thus giving compression and energy but not much development or complexity. Thus we don't find narrative features of longer formats (short stories, novels, epics), such as flashbacks, subplots, digressions, and elaborate descriptions. Jokes have a brief (or implied) setting, a very limited number of characters, a clear conflict, and a quick resolution—the so-called punch line, as if we'd been quickly struck by a hand. The appeals of stories in jokes include the following: the opening creates an interesting, hypothetical world that draws us in; the development of the plot creates mystery and suspense that keeps us guessing, and a resolution that surprises and pleases us, while also suggesting order (and sometimes justice). There are two exceptions to these descriptions: the shaggy dog story, which can be extended by internal repetition (even trying a listener's patience), and parodies that follow a given form, often quite lengthy. While some jokes are realistic, many cheerfully abandon norms of realism in favor of fantasy, whimsy, absurdity, and extravagance, although it's important that some realism gives at least an air of plausibility to the opening scene.

Earlier we discussed the Night Sea Journey, which has basic structure of stasis, chaos, and a new stasis; this format is useful for jokes about injury and sickness, which provide the chaotic middle portion. The resolution of a new stasis, however, can be of many sorts, including the agreement about the mistress of the corrupt Dr. and Mrs. Flynn and the contrasting outcomes for the Terrier and the Great Dane. As readers and hearers of jokes, we enjoy the sense of wholeness and order the brief narrative provides as well as, of course, clever humor. Narratives, even in very short forms, give a sense of order and control, and the rituals of sharing them allow teller and listener to agree, however subconsciously, that such order and control are good.

When we discussed Northrop Frye's division of stories, we focused on the desires of the central characters: if they are excluded from the community they wanted to join, the story is tragic, but if the character is included into the desired community, the story is comic. Sometimes the two basic myths are combined. In the parrot joke, the foul-mouthed bird is exiled from the man's society and almost frozen to death, tragically. When the man rescues the bird, restoring him to his society comically, the bird professes to be ready to adopt the local norms of speech. His wily, untrammeled side is still alive imaginatively, however, because he would like to know what extremes the turkey acted out before his (presumed) tragic punishment. Similarly, "In The Veterinarian's Waiting Room" presents a Terrier that (or who) does not fit into the genteel world of the mistresses and will be castrated—clearly tragic. The Great Dane figure is somewhat more complex. He is large, well-spoken, and, compared to the Terrier, a Dog of the World. He has had the good fortune that his sexual outburst occurred in private and was—magically and comically enough—well received. The trajectory of his narrative is positive: his medical treatment of nail trimming welcomes him to his comic community in his mistress' apartment, presumably for other sexual encounters, all versions—however strange—of the Green World.

The outcome of a story is not always comic, of course, and humor that shows conflict is often dark, sarcastic, even macabre.

A man was in a terrible industrial accident, and his genitals were ripped from his body, but saved by the paramedics and delivered to the hospital along with the patient.

The plastic surgeon put the genitals in a cooler and explained to the man and his wife that reattachment was now possible and, not only that, but a resizing was possible.

Since, however, insurance considered this cosmetic, it would not be covered. The prices would be as follows: small, $12,000; medium, $22,000; and large, $28,000.

The man was sure that small was out of the question, but that he couldn't decide between medium and large.

The doctor urged them to think about it overnight and give him their decision in the morning.

The next day the doctor comes to the hospital room and finds the wife smiling but the husband frowning.

"What did you decide?" he asks.

The man replied, "She'd rather remodel the kitchen."

We'll look more closely at humor that attacks through satire, sarcasm, or parody in Chapter Eight.

In Summary

Characters and story are the major structures in jokes. The characters give life to the events and invite our emotional interest. Some characters are quite odd, even absurd, as in the Great Dane and the hornswoggled Clem. Such oddity gives variety, exaggeration, and imaginative entertainment to us as readers or hearers and allows for dramatic presentation of emotions that we feel in lesser forms. Humorous jokes about sickness and illness typically move well beyond realistic stories of sick people we know or journalistic accounts of patients' medical breakthroughs. Such jokes play with norms of biology, medicine, and psychology through variations small, large, or hyperbolic. The dentist adjusting the chair for the woman who'd "rather have a baby" sounds practical according to crazy logic, but we know he would never say such a thing even as a joke. The playfulness of jokes allow us to exercise our imagination, admit to some of our hidden desires, and enjoy a ritual of sharing a joke with other people, even if such persons are only implied because we're reading the story on a page or on a computer screen. Well told jokes have basic stories that organize the events and build to a climax, usually with a surprise; a mood of tension and expectation suddenly pays off in a punch line that resolves the plot and gives another perspective. Sometimes there's a sense of poetic justice that reinforces implied social norms, as in Dr. and Mrs. Flynn. Sometimes the conclusion is just plan silly, as in the woman requesting a condom for a Camel. Even if the mood of the joke is strange, character and story give us a sense of wholeness and coherence, making a pleasing literary structure and a satisfying ritual as we hear or read it. During the time of the joke, or when we remember it later, we take a trip to the non-stressful Green World.

Chapter Eight

"Take This, You Moron!"

The Joys and Sorrows of Freudian Attacks

Betting On Drunks

From time to time the Emergency Room would receive a patient who was quite drunk. I don't mean happy and silly, talkative, singing, and/or making jokes. I mean totally wasted and unable to function beyond breathing, circulating blood, and other basic biochemical functions. It was useless to ask him (yes, usually a man, but not always) his name or address. Sometimes paramedics brought in such a patient from a car accident. Sometimes it was a so-called public drunk, someone picked up from a street or sidewalk.

In general, emergency personnel do not like patients who do themselves harm: driving too fast and causing an accident, not wearing a seat belt, or not wearing a motorcycle helmet—just to draw on the automotive world. They especially do not like when such risks endanger other, innocent people. In an Emergency Room there are plenty of people needing help already just from the ordinary absurdities of the world, so a crisis caused by a drug overdose or a game of Russian Roulette gone awry is not simply a distraction, it must take priority over other people. Suicide attempts are also disquieting, not only because of their (apparent) needlessness but also because of the implied mental turmoil that led to the event. I remember talking to a young man who had attempted to cut his wrists because his girlfriend was unfaithful. This patient had made the conventional slashes across his wrist, creating a mess in skin and the perpendicular tendon sheaths, with little real damage to the vasculature below that might have allowed him to bleed out and die. A doctor had to assess the damage then sew up all the damaged structures.

Some of the emotions among ER personnel that come forth with the arrival of a thoroughly intoxicated patient may include the following: anger at having to deal with this clearly avoidable event, pity toward a person who would mistreat himself this way, annoyance that this patient will take a certain amount of staff time, or disgust that humans can fall to such a state—for whatever reasons. Of course, ER folks know about addictions and other motivations, but a very drunk person coming into the ER is, from their point of view, unnecessary and disruptive to their work. And the spectacle of a fellow human being who has completely lost basic autonomy is, in itself, depressing.

So here's the ritual that indirectly expresses some of the emotions involved: it's a comedic ritual in the form of an office pool. A very drunk person on a midweek afternoon was, of course, an uncommon event. We did have a fair number of moderately intoxicated patients. Sometimes nurses would joke, "So, happy hour start a little early today?" and the patient would cheerfully agree. At this level of intoxication the patient and the nurses could kid around as fellow humans. But when a seriously intoxicated patient arrived, the mood was quite different, and there were no jokes between the nurse and the patient, who was, like the restrained patients we saw in Chapter Three, basically removed from society by being totally wasted. A nurse might, however, "start an envelope." Word would circulate, and ER personnel would stop by, take a quick look at the patient, write a number and initials on the envelope, and put a dollar inside. The patient's blood would go off to the lab for analysis, and—among other results—a blood alcohol level (BAL) would come back.

The BAL is expressed in milligrams of alcohol per 100 milliters of blood. A BAL of .10 means that one tenth of one percent (1/1000) of the blood content is alcohol. BAL is considered a good tool for legal enforcement because of its scientific nature (as opposed to, say, a policeman's observation). In my home state at the time, a BAL of 0.08 or above was enough for conviction for *driving under the influence* or DUI, but we often saw higher values in the ER. At 0.10, the drunk is typically noisy, acting strangely, and subject to mood swings; he has reduced reaction time, which makes him a danger on the highways. At 0.15 a person can have trouble walking. At 0.30, he can lose consciousness. Some die at 0.40. Because alcohol is a sedative, the intoxicated body and brain slow way down. At 0.50, breathing stops; many die.

One nurse had the reputation for extraordinary accuracy. She'd take a quick look and write her number—perhaps 0.18—and her initials. I often wondered whether other players would look at her guess and pick a nearby number. (That's how I, an outsider, might have played the game, but I never participated.) When the result came back from the lab, the winner's number was circled and the person notified. He or she would pocket all the dollars (perhaps $6, $8, or $10) and go on about usual business.

What did this strange game mean? I don't know what was in the mind of the nurses, and I'm not sure whether they themselves could explain the ideas and feelings involved. As I've thought about it, I've settled on the following interpretations.

The first level of meaning is a domestication of the bizarre through a game structure. The very drunk patient is a deviant and a threat to good social order: indeed he (or she) could have injured or killed someone with a vehicle. Further, he is at least a distraction and more likely a disruption to the ER since he'll need attention and care: he may vomit and aspirate, damaging his lungs, he may have serious injuries masked by the alcohol, he may have interactions with other drugs, and/or he may die. Or he may sober up enough to be loud and disruptive; he may try to hit a nurse. Through the lottery, the nurses reinforce their own comic community, reminding themselves that they are sober, well, and functioning, while the patient is none of these and therefore an outsider, a scapegoat.

The game itself is somewhere between a lottery (complete chance) and a rational contest using medical skill. The nurses are not picking random numbers; they take a look, get an impression, and compare to drunks they've seen before. In the larger culture, we have guessing games such as the number of jellybeans in a large jar, wine corks in a barrel, or fish in an aquarium tank. Some players make wild guesses, numbers plucked out of the air, but others make rough calculations based on geometric volume, a sample of one section, and so on. (Similarly, people who bet on horses, dogs, basketball, or poker often have their own "systems.") Whatever the strategy, the players participate in a game that they think they have a chance of winning, and they join in a shared social convention. As the nurses apply this structure to a drunken person, they objectify and isolate him, reclassifying him as a droll lab exhibit and, in a strange sense, domesticating him through their game. None of them, I think, do it for the small amount of money; they do it to deal emotionally with the intoxicated patient and to emphasize that they themselves are well.

The next idea, however, is paradoxical. When the jellybeans, or wine corks, or the fish are counted, the game is over, and life goes on. When the BAL comes back, it too is a specific number, but the underlying dilemma continues: the patient is still in the ER and very drunk. The domestication—such as it was—did not solve the absurdity brought into the space of the ER. In this sense, the game is doomed. Another reading, therefore, is that the bets are scornful gestures that express the anger of the nurses who cannot immediately treat and heal this man who is dangerous to himself and to others. The game, then, can be understood as a set of attacks on him, vengeful attempts to reduce him to a number, and, because these attacks are futile, they are indirect expressions of both anger and frustration.

FROM THE WORLD OF JOKES

What is 18 inches long and hangs in front of an asshole?
A stethoscope

⚕   ⚕   ⚕

The CEO of an HMO dies and goes to Saint Peter's Gate. Saint Peter looks over his record and says, "Well, it looks like a pretty good life. A few indiscretions, some greed, some mistreatment of your lowest-paid employees, but on the whole a hard-working life that merits acceptance into heaven."

And the CEO says, "Oh boy, that's really wonderful. What a relief!"

And Saint Peter says, "Yes, but you can stay only for three days."

⚕   ⚕   ⚕

The latest in mental health includes this advice for recovering from a rough day. You won't need drink, pills, or television. Simply follow the easy instructions in their numbered order:

1. Picture yourself near a deep pool of a pleasant stream.

2. Hear the birds softly chirping and feel the gentle breezes.

3. Enjoy the fact that no one knows you are here in your secret place.

4. Revel in the feeling that you are completely away from the ordinary world.

5. Hear the soft murmurings of the stream as it enters the pool.

6. Enjoy the clarity of the water as you look down into the pool.

7. The water is so wonderfully clear that you can easily make out the face of the person you are holding underwater.

These three jokes, even in very short compass, manage to attack a doctor, a CEO, and an enemy of the listener's/reader's choice. How are we to understand such verbal attacks?

In his *Jokes and Their Relation to the Unconscious* (1905; *Der Witz und Seine Beziehung zum Unbewussten*), Sigmund Freud spoke of many of the features we have been discussing: economy of jokes, play with language as pleasurable in suggesting freedom, childlike delight in absurdity, characters who are caricatures, and rebellion against authority. At half a dozen points, he sees similarities between jokes and dreams, about which he wrote extensively in *The Interpretation of Dreams* (1900): both forms of mental activity reveal hidden urges and desires from the unconscious; both are expressions of our deepest selves that emerge despite the repressive structures of rational thought (the super ego) and society (which has helped to construct the super ego).[1]

The focus for this chapter is Freud's argument that some jokes are tendentious—that is, they have an agenda or hidden argument, particularly through hostile attacks. Such attacks, through parody, satire, or invective, can be aimed at persons, ideas, social structures, or society's repressions in general. Speaking about jokes, he wrote, "They make possible the satisfaction of an instinct (whether lustful or hostile) in the face of an obstacle that stands in its way," an obstacle such as taboo. Writing in a formal Vienna around 1900, Freud had given up hope: "The repressive activity of civilization brings it about that primary possibilities of enjoyment, which have now, however, been repudiated by the censorship in us, are lost to us" (p. 101).

Today, norms of speech and mass media are much freer with lustful or hostile instincts (indeed too free, for some tastes). Specifically, humor about medicine, health, and mortality is now relatively free to express some of our deepest urges, often through attacks on persons, ideas, or institutions that to us seem unfair, absurd, or downright evil. At the same time, there is often a mirroring, in the sense that our attacks on outward targets often draw on our inner uncertainties and fears. Many of the jokes in this chapter illustrate this dual movement, an outward attack and an inner turmoil.

ATTACKING THROUGH HUMOR

Some attacks are gentle, some ferocious. Let's start with a relatively gentle joke:

> There was a terrible auto wreck, and people burst out of houses, offices, and shops to run to the car which had smashed into a tree. One of the first to reach the scene was a small woman, but a large man who came next lifted her up by her shoulders and set her aside, saying "Out of the way, little lady. I've had first aid training!"

"Well, good for you," said she. "And when you get to the part about calling a doctor, I'll be standing right here."

"Good for you" is, of course, sarcastic, since her own "goodness" of many years of medical training and experience far outweighs his. There's a slightly harder edge to her ironic statement that she'd stand there waiting while the victims suffer. Finally, there's a battle in the war of the sexes: the large man touched her without her permission (technically the crime of battery) and moved her aside, as if she were insignificant; she cannot counter by physical force, but she can attack with words that indicate her superior medical status and social position. After all, she could say, "Hey, buddy, I'm a doctor, and I'm taking charge here until the paramedics arrive," but the joke prefers a more arch comment that shames the man who acted in such a chauvinistic, improper way.

Other jokes imputing male inferiority are cast more specifically in medical terms:

> Q. Why is psychoanalysis a lot quicker for men than for women?
> A. Because when it's time to go back to his childhood, he's already there.

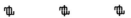

A woman walks into a pharmacy and asks the pharmacist for some arsenic. He asks, "What for?"

She says, "I want to kill my husband."

He says, "Sorry, I can't do that."

She then reaches into her handbag and pulls out a photo of her husband in bed with the pharmacist's wife and hands it to him.

He says, "You didn't tell me you had a prescription."

The pharmacist, we may assume, feels immediate hatred and urge for revenge, but nonetheless he makes a matter-of-fact utterance using the euphemistic medical term "prescription." The joke attacks his professional ethics that he professed to hold by having him abandon them in a heartbeat.

A man goes to a shrink and says, "Doctor, my wife is unfaithful to me. Every evening, she goes to Larry's bar and picks up men. In fact, she sleeps with anybody who asks her! I'm going crazy. What do you think I should do?"

"Relax," says the Doctor, "take a deep breath and calm down. I understand the pain you must be going through. But first, why don't you just tell me, exactly where is Larry's bar?"

This joke reflects our inner fears of betrayal and loss of a spouse's fidelity, but also betrayal by medical professionals. As in the pharmacist joke, the doctor here mouths professional language but quickly acts on his own sanguine and selfish urges.

A devoted wife spent her life taking care of her husband. Now he was in an ICU, slipping in and out of a coma. She spent days at the hospital, faithfully watching and comforting him when he was lucid. One day, he motioned for her to come closer and whispered in her ear, "When I had the car wreck, you were there to support me. When my business failed, you were there to support me. When we lost our house, you supported me. When my health failed, you supported me. I've been thinking it all over."

"Yes, dear?"

"I believe you bring me bad luck!"

At a literary level, perhaps we enjoy the reversal of moods and the way the wife is tricked. At a subconscious level, we are reminded of tensions between husbands and wives, dynamics of blaming, and other irrational behavior. The harshness of this joke may remind us that the word "sarcasm" has a Greek root *sarkazein*, meaning to tear flesh. Indeed, that this man is so utterly awful to his wife may allow us to feel pride that we aren't so bad. The joke reminds us that there is evil in the world and, in the telling of it, encapsulates it.

Sometimes the battle of the sexes is a little lighter in mood.

A husband and wife, both 65, sometimes bicker. Today, she goes to the doctor for a check-up.

Back home, her husband badgers her for all the details.

"I'm just terrific," she temporizes. "He said, among other things, that I have the legs of a 30-year-old."

"Yeah, I'll bet."

"Not only that, but the breasts of a 23-year old."

"Yeah, I'll bet."

"And the waist of a teenager!"

"Yeah, whatever. Did he say anything about your 65-year-old ass?"

"Why no: your name didn't come up!"

And here's a similar joke, again with word play but with higher stakes:

A husband and wife were talking over the possibilities of serious illness and how extensive medical treatment should be.

The husband said, "Well, all things considered, I think that I do not wish to live in a vegetative state, with fluids dripping into me, all dependent on some machine. If I ever get like that, I'd want you to pull the plug."

Ever attentive, his wife stood up, unplugged the TV, then went to the refrigerator and threw out all his beer.

Neither that joke nor the following need comment or explanation.

A man visits his therapist and complains that, once again, he has not been able to be assertive in self-disclosure and has failed, once again, to say what he really means.

"Tell me about it, won't you?" invites the therapist.

"Well, I said to my wife, 'You really annoy me.'"

"That seems pretty direct to me. How is that a failure?"

"Don't you see? What I really wanted to say was 'You've destroyed my life, you castrating bitch!'"

DOCTORS AND SEX

During an office visit, Mr. Jones awaits Dr. White's diagnosis.

Dr. White says, "I've got good news and bad news. Which do you want first?"

"Well, I guess we'd better get the bad news over with first."

"Ok, the bad news is that you have an aggressive cancer."

"Oh my God. That's terrible. Whatever can the good news be?"

"You know the tall nurse with the big breasts? I'm having an affair with her!"

In this cynical joke, there are two attacks. The doctor attacks the patient by promising good news (presumably regarding his care, perhaps an easy, successful treatment for his kind of cancer) but delivering an irrelevant comment about his own sex life. There can be no justification for such an attack of course, which leads us to the second attack: the joke criticizes Dr. White, who is shown to be cruel, greedy, self-absorbed, and immoral. If we laugh, it's because we recognize (and dislike) the asymmetrical relationship of the overly sanguine doctor who is in the world of the well but who has just assigned to Mr. Jones to the world of the sick. The joke draws on our hatred of manipulative power relationships, especially if we're in the powerless position.

Patient, post-surgery: "Doctor, doctor! I can't feel anything."

Doctor: "Now, now, don't worry: that's perfectly normal in a case like yours. We cut off your hands."

We saw this joke in Chapter Six, emphasizing the images. Here we may comment on the Freudian attack. The patient—in a most vulnerable state—is attacked by the cruel doctor, and the doctor is attacked by the joke as taking advantage in the doctor-patient power relationship to toy with the patient. He may even be a mutilator without medical cause. The pun on "feel" makes the double behanding plausible within the joke, but it also suggests that it is the doctor who can't "feel" what the patient's experience is and act appropriately.

A man and a woman exchange glances at a bar; he moves to her table and they have more drinks. Conversation goes well, and she invites him to her apartment. They arrive there. In her bedroom he takes off his shirt then steps through the bathroom door and washes his hands. He takes off his trousers and washes his hands.

"You must be a dentist," she says.

"Why, yes, I am," he says, surprised. "How did you know?"

"Easy. You keep washing your hands."

"Oh, of course."

One thing leads to another and they make love.

Afterwards, she says, "You must be a very good dentist."

And, quite full of himself from the evening's developments, he replies, "You bet I am. How did you figure that out?"

"Easy. I didn't feel a thing."

This strange joke satirizes the dentist in two ways: he's compulsively germ-free and also incapable of giving sexual pleasure to a female. It's a harsh joke, giving a punful, post-coital meaning to the dental cliché, "you won't feel a thing." As many patients (myself included) have an unreasonable dread of dentists, we seem to enjoy an attack on this dentist as revenge for our fears. Dental work suggests a violation of our privacy, a threat of pain, and an opportunity for injury or change in our appearance. Dentists know all this of course (they have teeth also) and must work under exacting conditions (small space, nervous patients, and medicolegal contexts). Dentists who understand nervous patients do their best to put them at ease.

Another joke adds male-female conflict:

Mrs. Jones is in the dentist's chair. He approaches her and says, "Open, please." She opens her mouth and, as she does so, she reaches out and grabs his genitals.

"Hey, watch it!" he exclaims.

"Let's just agree," she says, "that neither of us shall hurt the other."

Perhaps we admire her attempt to achieve a symmetrical relationship in a realm that is strongly asymmetrical.

We leave the dentist's office for this joke, which ends unexpectedly.

Doctor Donald had slept with one of his patients for the very first time in his career. Although there was some joy in the coupling, he felt very guilty about it. No matter how much he tried to forget about it, he just couldn't.

But every once in a while he'd hear an internal, reassuring voice in his head that said: "Donald, don't cry about it. You aren't the first medical practitioner to sleep with one of their patients and you won't be the last. And you're single. You were responsible and used precautions. You both enjoyed it. Just let it go!"

But invariably another voice in his head would bring him back to reality, whispering, "Donald, that was very bad, against all professional regulations; not only was that one of your patients, but also—it must be said—you are a veterinarian."

This joke leads us to imagine the possibilities of Donald's partner, all of them very much taboo. Like the Great Dane in the Waiting Room joke, Donald has had interspecies experience, but the Great Dane appeared to be a sanguine and wise character, while Donald is attacked here as a pervert of sorts. The two voices create the ambiguity: the first allowing us to imagine a human-human sexual act, but the second voice surprises us by indirectly but clearly suggesting the animality of his sexual experience. The joke attacks the veterinarian and perhaps us too as we imaginatively consider his possible partners.

DOCTORS AND MONEY

Q. What's the definition of a doctor?

A. Someone who kills your ills with pills, then kills you with his bills.

Ah, money, a clear symbol of power and control! We feel that it's bad enough being sick or injured, but then we must also make payments at further cost to our social power (not to mention time waiting, lost work, or losses to family and social life). And we may even suspect that our money goes to make doctors wealthy and fatten the bottom lines of conniving insurance companies.

Here's an attack upon not only the cupidity of a dentist but his cruelty as well.

Mr. Smith has a toothache. The dentist examines the tooth, takes an X-ray, and says, "I'm sorry, Mr. Smith, but this tooth is so decayed that there's nothing I can do to save it. I'm afraid it must come out."

"Oh, no," he says. "And how much will that cost?"

"The standard extraction fee is $300."

"THREE HUNDRED DOLLARS for just a few minutes work?" he cries out.

"That's right, that's the usual fee. But, you know, I can extract it very slowly if you'd prefer."

⚖   ⚖   ⚖

Two men are playing golf.

One says, "My doctor told me to avoid stress."

"Good idea. I suppose that's why you're out playing golf today?"

"Oh sure, but the main thing is that I don't open any of his bills."

Jokes that attack doctors in terms of money illustrate several human failings. First, of course, is envy and jealousy; wouldn't it be nice to make a very large income such as doctors receive? Second, is general ignorance about the debts doctors run up while in medical school, the high payments that they make for malpractice insurance, and other costs of running a business (staff, medical transcription, billing, weekend coverage), as well as the long hours they work and the continuous stress they experience. The stress has many sources: personal demands for excellence, institutional requirements, ethical and legal constraints, patients who don't improve even with the best of care, and so on. How many jealous people would, in fact, trade for a doctor's life? The third human failing is a reductive judgment that money is the main thing that matters for doctors, a pervasive symbol in a consumer society that values cars and houses, expensive travel, and "net worth." In such jokes attacking doctors, we project upon them our complicity in a consumer culture. In fact, medical personnel typically care a lot about their patients and the health of society as a whole.

Lawyers Have Their Turn

There is sometimes conflict between doctors and lawyers, often because lawyers represent clients bringing lawsuits against doctors for malpractice. It may also be said that medicine and law often attract very bright, highly motivated, and competitive people who sometimes rub each other the wrong way. (Yes, that's an idiom that has the buried image of stroking an animal's coat.)

There have been numerous lawyer jokes over the last few decades; many are presented and analyzed in Marc Galanter's book, *Lowering the Bar*.[2] (He has versions of the two following jokes on page 213 and page 207.)

Q. What's the definition of a tragedy?

A. A bus full of lawyers going over a cliff with two seats empty.

There's a medical joke that is even more hostile:

A woman is visiting her OB/GYN. After a routine examination, the doctor tells her everything is fine and that they're finished.

She hesitates, however, and mutters that there is something that's troubling her.

The doctor kindly encourages her to ask her question.

"Well...I'm so embarrassed to ask this, because I thought I knew the answer...."

"That's perfectly all right," the doctor soothes, "any question is just fine here."

"Well, OK, then...my husband has been somewhat persistent about some sexual experimentation, and I need to know...well, can you become pregnant from anal intercourse?"

"I'm so glad you asked that," replies the doctor, "because there's a lot of misunderstanding about that."

"Really?"

"Yes. And in fact, you can become pregnant from that activity."

"You're sure?"

"Yes, of course. Where do you think lawyers come from?"

Heathcare Institutions

And now a public service announcement parody:

The Centers for Disease Control and Prevention have released a list of symptoms of bird flu. If you experience any of the following, please seek medical treatment immediately:

1. *High fever*
2. *Congestion*
3. *Nausea*
4. *Fatigue*
5. *Aching in the joints*
6. *An irresistible urge to crap on someone's windshield.*

Ah, the glories of nonparallelism! The punch line has two attacks. The first is the personification (avianification?) of us as birds, as if we were anxious to relieve ourselves on cars—or any other target. Like monkeys hurling their feces at startled visitors to the zoo, we might crap on anything that we hate or simply on anything at all, a wonderfully cathartic thought, especially for people who "watch their tongue," "count to ten before speaking when angry," "keep their hands to themselves," "manage their anger," and so forth. The joke acknowledges our unconscious urges to act in uncivilized ways—a common Freudian notion—and places it at the animal level of birds. Filth from the sky is an annoyance so grotesque, so gratuitous, so unnecessary, that we're glad to have it identified as a disease that, according to the joke, Our Government is now expertly fighting! The last attack, of course, is in the parody of a CDCP warning, suggesting that it is crazy and therefore ineffective—as in the catch phrase, "close enough for government work!"

Hospitals, Doctors' Offices

For decades people have complained about hospital food and nurses waking up patients in order to administer sleeping pills, two instances of institutional control. Here are two jokes that attack such things.

Mr. Jones was sitting on a hospital bed, fully dressed, with a suitcase nearby. The nurse arrived with a wheelchair and said, "You'll need to go in this."

"But I'm perfectly fine," he said.

"No ifs ands or buts. Hospital policy. Get in. Now!" she ordered.

He did so. She wheeled him out of the room and down the hall to the elevator.

While descending in the elevator, the nurse asked, "And just where are we meeting your wife?"

"Got me," he said. "As far as I know she's still upstairs in the bathroom, changing out of her hospital gown."

☙　　☙　　☙

Mr. Smith goes to the doctor's office to pick up some test results for his wife. The nurse says, "You're going to have to speak with our office manager," and leads him to that office.

The manager says, "Mr. Smith, we can't definitively provide you with the results because there's been a mix-up."

"Really?"

"Well, yes. There were two Mrs. Smiths in that day and their samples became confused. Either way, however, it's not good."

"Whatever do you mean?"

"One Mrs. Smith tested positive for Alzheimer's, while the other tested positive for AIDS."

"Oh, no! That's terrible. Either way!"

"Yes, very bad."

"We'd better run the tests again to see which she has," says Mr. Smith.

"That makes sense, but your HMO will pay for such tests only once a year, and you've had yours."

"What?"

"But we did call the HMO, and they thought of another solution."

"Oh, good! What is it?"

"You drop your wife off on the edge of town. If she remembers her way home, don't sleep with her."

This is a thoroughly sarcastic joke, ascribing cruelty to the HMO and the complicity of the doctor's office. Yet patients who have battled faceless bureaucrats and number crunchers from HMOs, insurance companies, billing departments of hospitals, and the like may appreciate the joke's attack on all such, showing them to be inept and uncaring. Sometimes the symbolism is monetary; institutions refuse to pay (or pay only fractionally) for medical treatment. We resent such power of a large, anonymous entity over us, an entity with complex, even mysterious rules. Furthermore, it feels like robbery: the resource that could pay does not, and so it's we who become liable.

HMOs and Insurance Companies

Here is an elaborate parody of a question-and-answer series that might appear in a newspaper column or a brochure at a hospital. Once again, a writer has taken the time and talent to attack the concept of an HMO, posting this on the Web.

Explanations Of Medical Policies

Q. What does HMO stand for?

A. This is actually a variation of the phrase, "HEY MOE." Its roots go back to a concept pioneered by Moe of the Three Stooges, who discovered that a patient could be made to forget about the pain in his foot if he was poked hard enough in the eyes.

Q. I just signed up for Medical Insurance. How difficult will it be to choose the doctor I want?

A. Just slightly more difficult than choosing your parents. Your insurer will provide you with a book listing all the doctors in the plan.

These doctors basically fall into two categories: (1) those who are no longer accepting new patients, and (2) those who will see you but are no longer participating in the plan. But don't worry; the remaining doctor who is still in the plan and accepting new patients has an office just a half-day's drive away, and a diploma from a Third World country.

Q. Do all diagnostic procedures require pre-certification?

A. No. Only those you need.

Q. Can I get coverage for my preexisting conditions?

A. Certainly, as long as they don't require any treatment.

Q. What happens if I want to try alternative forms of medicine?

A. You'll need to find alternative forms of payment.

Q. My pharmacy plan only covers generic drugs, but I need the name brand. I tried the generic medication, but it gave me a stomach ache. What should I do?

A. Poke yourself in the eye.

Q. What if I'm away from home and I get sick?

A. You really shouldn't do that.

Q. I think I need to see a specialist, but my doctor insists he can handle my problem. Can a general practitioner really perform a heart transplant right in his office?

A. Hard to say, but considering that all you're risking is the $20 co-payment, there's no harm in giving him a shot at it.

Q. Will health care be different in the next century?

A. No. But if you call right now, you might get an appointment by then.

MEDICARE

An elderly couple arrive by taxi at a doctor's office. They ask the receptionist to be seen by the doctor together to discuss "a private matter."

Noting their different last names, the tactful receptionist agrees to their request.

The man and woman wait in an examining room. The doctor enters and asks what he can do for them.

"Well, we're not married, but we're deeply in love. Lately, however, we've been having some problems of sexual incompatibility."

The doctor asks some questions, looks them over briefly, and says, "I'm not finding much here. Tell you what: there's a room at the end of the hall that you could use for sex. Give it a try and then tell me more exactly what the problem is."

They oldsters agree and go to the room.

Thirty minutes later they come out, pink and happy.

They report to the doctor that things went pretty well today, but they weren't sure of future encounters.

A week later they're back and go through the same routine.

A week after that, they're back. The doctor is getting suspicious. "What's going on with you two?"

"Well, the nursing home won't let us have sex there, and the Holiday Inn costs $89. We can come here for our $10 co-pay and Medicare picks up the rest!"

CATHARSIS

As mentioned earlier, cartharsis is a good old Aristotelian term perhaps never improved upon, even by Freud. In Aristotle's *Poetics*, catharsis meant the cleansing of emotions through watching a tragedy on the stage. Aristotle's scientific mind sensed that emotions were bad things and they needed to be purged. Watching a tragedy on stage or screen can arouse feelings of loss, sadness, or betrayal that we have individually experienced. If we weep, it is both for those characters and for hurts we ourselves have suffered. In the public culture of happy-happy America, many of these hurts stay buried, repressed by taboo and images of "being strong." We have phrases like, "Shake it off," "Tough guys don't cry," and (a favorite from Westerns) "It's only a flesh wound." Indeed, because Americans are *supposed* to be so happy and healthy we may feel inadequate or cowardly by admitting that we feel pain, betrayal, or terror. Humor is one relatively safe way to deal with such emotions, although it may only mention them without going much deeper. In medical settings, we may experience fear and/or anger that doctors should see us intimately in an asymmetrical relationship, that we should bare our weaknesses to them, and, finally, that they have no absolute power to cure us and are sometimes helpless themselves.

In Summary

Attacking humor heals us, first, by representing things we dislike, fear, and even hate and, second, by allowing us to know that other people have also been troubled by such things. The humor can be as simple as name-calling (Crispy Critter, Cancer Sucks), or as complicated as an elaborate parody, as in "Explanations of Medical Policies" just seen. Derisive laughter provides a ritual of revenge, a catharsis (however temporary) of emotions such as fear, loss, insecurity, betrayal, even terror that can be part of illness and healthcare. Finally, behind each attack, there is a positive value: the jokes affirm that it's better not to be burned or not to have cancer, and it's better to have humane medical policies. In a roundabout way, attacking humor typically affirms basic personal and social values, as well as providing entertainment and the inventiveness of imagery, language, character, and story.

Chapter Nine

Aging and Death

We're All in the Same Damn Boat

NOONTIME CONFERENCE: A BAD CASE OF THE TMBs

Some family practice residents were getting their food before their noontime conference.

"Hey, what's up with Mr. Sullivan?" one asked another.

"Oh, there's not much I can do for him; it's a really bad case of the TMBs."

"Oh, that's too bad."

"With secondary PPP?" asked another.

"Absolutely."

"Indicating TOBAS?" said a third.

"A most definite indication."

"So he's pretty well screwed," said one of them.

"Yes, and so am I."

To an outsider this sounds like a "curbside consult," or a casual exchange of medical views about a patient—that is, up to the last two lines, about being "screwed." Abbreviations by initials are commonplace in medical speech, case presentations, and charts: COPD means chronic obstructive pulmonary disease; CHF means congestive heart failure, STD means sexually transmitted disease, ETOH means alcohol abuse, and so on. In the conversation above, however, the initials are satiric, because they refer to slang phrases, not technical concepts from medicine. Here's the key:

    TMBs = Too Many Birthdays

    PPP = Piss-Poor Protoplasm

    TOBAS = Take Out Back And Shoot

Some of these have been around for a long time while others, like most slang, have come and gone. (Note: the dialogue is not a transcript of an actual event but rather a conflation of several comments.)

We have three levels of meaning: (1) the surface level of the initials bandied about, appearing as medical terminology, (2) the secondary meanings that the initials stand for, a satiric code among a particular community, and (3) an indirect, implicit reference to the limits of medicine, because Mr. Sullivan is at an advanced age and his body is inevitably breaking down. The subterfuge of the code allows the resident doctors (typically in their twenties or thirties) to break the taboo in this culture that we don't speak of the inevitability of death. But their verbal play does not go deeply into this difficult subject. Part of their dilemma, of course, is the inability of medicine to *cure the illnesses* of such patients and, beyond that, the inability of much of medical culture to *heal patients into death*. Medicine—as currently conceived with *cure* as its main priority—is ultimately and necessarily a failure when dying and death are concerned, and physicians are, therefore, failures as well. Perhaps the satiric terminology hides resentment, anger, and despair about medicine's limits. When I observed in a Family Medicine Residency, I was struck by the pain the young physicians felt when their aging patients were inevitably dying.

Aging and death are very common themes in the oral tradition, especially when they are perceived as threats to cultural values of youthful appearance, high energy, and infinite promise. Worse yet, aging and death are conditions that no amount of money, success, or medicine can surmount. Thus we have an intractable irony: we prize choice, freedom, proactivity, projects, goals, agency, autonomy, and achievements, but we know we are doomed to a lifespan with a definite (if unknown) limit. Furthermore, we may have serious forms of weakness and debility before our deaths. We may want to feel, with British Victorian William Ernest Henley that "I am the master of my fate: / I am the captain of my soul," but deep down we know it just ain't so.

Within the pervasive theme of aging versus agency, there is once again the common theme of sexual power, a marker of our health and well-being. Vital youth, we seem to assume, is always eager for and capable of sex, while old people obviously have lost both capacity and interest. Much advertising is aimed at youth, in hopes of having life-long consumers of services and products, and such advertising has used sex to "turn our heads toward" a product or service (the meanings of the Latin roots *ad* and *vert*). Clearly, if youth is good, old age is bad. In some jokes, old people are scapegoated as stupid and worthless, in part because they are no longer wage earners building the capitalist kingdom. Besides, they are just one step away from death, a difficult mystery for secular culture.

Some of these attitudes are changing as the population gets older and as aging people have more and more agency, influence, and even economic power. Thus we find some jokes that are playful in acknowledging changing bodies and capacities, while other jokes are harsher, attacking in a Freudian sense.

From The World Of Jokes

Signs Of Menopause
1. You sell your home heating system at a yard sale.
2. You write your kids' names on their foreheads.
3. You change your underwear after a sneeze.

☫   ☫   ☫

An older couple is lying in bed one morning, slowly waking up. He takes her hand gently, but she says, "Don't touch me."

"Why not?" he asks.

"Because I'm dead."

"Whatever are you talking about! You're as alive as I am."

"I'm definitely dead."

"You're not dead. I can see you, smell you, even touch you. So why are you saying this?"

"Because I woke up this morning and nothing hurts!"

☫   ☫   ☫

Researchers from the American Medical Association have made a pivotal discovery that some patients may benefit from receiving blood from chickens rather than from humans. Such treatment tends to make the men cocky and the women lay better.

Aging

As the Baby Boomers (some seventy-eight million strong) careen into Middle Age and Beyond, concerns with aging show up in numerous jokes, many flying around the Internet. A person born in 1946 was amazed in 2011 to find himself or herself sixty-five years old, a common age for retirement. He or she grew up in the fifties, a time (for many) of security and wealth. Many Boomers have had successful lives, at least as defined with accumulation of material things and wealth in general. Many knew peace for much of their lives as well as the end of the Cold War. Many have gone to high school or college reunions, often giving some attention to how they look beforehand. At such reunions, they saw a wide variety of health and well-being. Some of their peers still looked good. Some had aged considerably. Some were dead. No matter how much money, how many possessions, how much status a Boomer has, he or she gets older. In a society that prizes the attributes of youth, there is a pervasive neurosis about aging, and humor is the predictable and necessary result.

At this writing I'm in my late sixties, and family members and friends—even from grade school—who are similarly old all send me jokes about dilemmas of aging. It's also true that some of my friends from high school and college have died in the past five years. Many people have said some version of this: "As bad as it is, getting old beats *the alternative*," a euphemistic reference to our inevitable deaths.

A Range of Declining Capacities

Jokes touch on several declining capacities of the elderly.

Old Is When

1. Going bra-less pulls all the wrinkles out of your face.
2. Getting a little action means "I don't need fiber today."
3. "Getting lucky" means you find your car in the parking lot.
4. An all-nighter means not getting up to pee.

Remember, once you get over the hill, you'll begin to pick up speed.

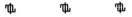

An elderly gentleman had serious hearing problems for many years.

He went to the doctor, and the doctor was able to have him fitted for a set of hearing aids that allowed him to hear perfectly.

The elderly gentleman went back in a month to the doctor and the doctor said, "Your hearing is perfect. Your family must be really pleased that you can hear again."

The gentleman replied, "Oh, I haven't told my family yet. I just sit around and listen to the conversations. I've changed my will three times!"

An old man needs surgery; fortunately for him, his son is a surgeon renowned for the necessary procedure. The old man makes the arrangements and travels to the son's hospital.

They're visiting before the operation, and the old man says, "Don't be nervous, son. Just do your best. And remember, if anything happens to me, your mother is going to come to live with you and your wife."

Two elderly gentlemen from a retirement center were sitting on a bench under a tree when one turns to the other and says: "Slim, I'm eighty-three years old now and I'm just full of aches and pains. I know you're about my age. How do you feel?"

Slim says, "I feel just like a newborn baby."

"Really? Like a new-born baby?"

"Yep. No hair, no teeth, and I think I just wet my pants."

֎   ֎   ֎

A group of senior citizens are sitting in a Florida senior center.

"My arthritis is so bad, I can barely hold this glass of iced tea," says one.

"Yeah, it's a crime," says another. "And I can barely see my glass."

"My pills for blood pressure make me dizzy," contributes a third.

"Ain't it a bear. I can't turn my head anymore," says another.

"Well, I guess that's what's getting old is all about," says the first.

"I guess so," says the second. "Thank heavens we can all still drive!"

The last joke makes light of some very real automotive risks. I lived in Florida for some thirty years, and aging drivers were a common topic for conversation, especially when there were newspaper stories about oldsters driving cars through store windows, off sea walls, and over bridges that were in the process of opening.

Loss of Mental Faculties

A dapper elderly man enters an upscale bar. He's wearing a blazer, a tie, and pressed slacks. His hair is neat, and he smells of aftershave lotion.

He sits down at the bar next to an elderly woman. They smile at each other.

He leans toward her, and asks, "Tell me, do I come here often?"

With the aging of our population, loss of mental function is more and more a threat, and our jokes about senility illustrate our worry about such deficits.

Two elderly people lived in a Florida mobile home park: he, a widower, and she, a widow. They had been good friends for a number of years.

One evening there was a community supper at the activity center. The two sat across a table from each other, exchanging admiring glances. Over dessert, the man said to her, "Will you marry me?"

She finished her dessert thoughtfully and took a swallow of coffee.

"Yes," she said, "I will."

They shared a brief hug then departed in different directions to their respective trailers.

The next morning he woke up in a state of confusion. Did she say yes or no? He had no idea. He ransacked his mind for details, but nothing became clear.

He was embarrassed and nervous, but he picked up the phone and called her. Taking his time, he explained that he didn't remember as well as he once did and that he was embarrassed to have to ask, "What did you say when I asked you to marry me. Was it yes or no?"

"Oh, I said yes," she replied. "I said I would be so glad to marry you."

"Oh that's great!" he said.

And she said, "And I'm so glad you called, because, to tell the truth, I couldn't remember who had asked me."

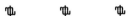

An elderly couple had dinner at another couple's house. After eating, the wives left the table and went into the kitchen. The two husbands chatted at the table. One said, "Last night we went to a new restaurant and had a wonderful meal. I would recommend it very highly."

The other man said, "Great, and what was the name of that place?"

The first man thought and thought and finally said, "Say, what's the name of that flower you give to a sweetheart, smells nice, but lots of thorns?"

"You mean a rose?"

"Yes, just so," he said. He then turned toward the kitchen and yelled out, "Rose, what's the name of that restaurant we went to last night?"

LIMINAL SPACES, FOR EXAMPLE, NURSING HOMES

Nursing homes are a common but difficult subject for jokes, especially if there are memories of "old folks homes" that were poorly run places for old people who were abandoned and mistreated. Whatever the name, such facilities may be seen as a liminal place, a way station between life and death, especially when patients have no realistic chance of recovery and return to their own homes. Modern retirement homes typically have three levels of care: independent living, assisted living, and a medical center (which may have a dementia section or wing). In her final years, my mother lived in such a place and passed through all three levels.

I recall a medical wing where my mother, at ninety-two, was failing. After our first visit, my wife and I stood in the parking lot, hugged each other, and cried. We were overwhelmed by the sight of many moribund people sitting in wheelchairs because this culture does not show these folks in movies, in print, or on TV and also because it was likely to be my mother's fate. It might be ours as well.

Because many of us are unfamiliar with the sights, sounds, smells, even elevated temperatures of nursing homes, we have no realistic images of them. Instead we have unrealistic images from the world of jokes, which, nonetheless, realistically represent some of our hopes, fears, doubts, even anger. We recall from Chapter Six the joke about Viagra to keep a male patient in bed and the joke about the nurses not allowing a patient to pass gas. We can see these as attacks on the indignities of being in such places. A bumper sticker sarcastically comments on family dynamics and our fears of abandonment: *Be kind to your children: they'll choose your nursing home.*

The next two jokes are somewhat different.

There's a commotion at the door of the rec room at the retirement center as elderly Eunice bursts into the room.

She holds a clenched fist high in the air and yells out, "Hey! Anyone who can guess what I have in my hand can have sex with me tonight!"

As in most retirement centers, the room is mostly filled with women, but the handful of men look over, some interested, some not.

One man calls out, "An elephant?"

Eunice replies, "Close enough!"

⚘   ⚘   ⚘

A small energetic woman is running up and down the halls of her nursing home. At each door, she flips up the hem of her nightgown and calls out, "Supersex!"

When she reaches the lounge at the end of the hall she approaches an old man in a wheelchair. She flips up her nightgown and calls out, "Supersex!"

The man thinks carefully for a moment, scratches his head, and says, "I think I'll take the soup."

These two jokes project, somewhat extravagantly, our hopes that we may have sexual energy, even when we are in retirement homes.

DEATH

Predictably enough, death is a topic fraught with emotions and meanings, a subject for comic treatment in jokes. The ones below proceed, very roughly, from harsh to playful.

Mildred was a ninety-four-year-old woman who was particularly despondent over the recent death of her husband, Earl. She decided that she would just kill herself and join him in death. Thinking that it would be best to get it over with quickly, she took out Earl's old Army pistol and made the decision to shoot herself in the heart, since it was so badly broken.

Not wanting to miss the vital organ and become a vegetable and burden to someone, she called her doctor's office to inquire as to just exactly where the heart would be on a woman.

The doctor said, "Your heart would be just below your left breast."

Later that night, Mildred was admitted to the hospital with a gunshot wound to her knee.

FAMOUS LAST WORDS

"You said these are the good mushrooms, right?"

"I wonder what this button does?"

"Isn't this bear cub cute. I wonder where the mother is?"

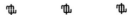

A woman goes into the newspaper office to prepare a death notice for her husband. She is alarmed to learn that the cost is a dollar per word, and thinks of the shortest way to put the news. Finally she writes on the form, "John Brown died."

The clerk says, "Well, that's terse and efficient, all right, but I'm afraid we have a seven-word minimum."

The woman thinks a moment, then completes her formulation: "John Brown died; golf clubs for sale."

Waiter: Are you ready to order, sir?

Mr. Smith: Just about. I do have one question.

Waiter: Yes?

Mr. Smith: How do you prepare your chickens?

Waiter: Oh nothing special, really. We just tell them they're going to die.

Three guys are drinking and talking about getting old.

"Hey, you know, when it's all said and done," one says, "You'll be lying there in your casket, you know, in your suit. And what would you like folks to say about you as they pass by?"

And Frank says, "Well, I guess that I was a good family man and did my job well and kept up the house and yard."

And Jim says, "Yeah, stuff like that, and I was a good Christian and helped out in the neighborhood. What about you?"

"Oh heck, that's easy. I'd like them to say, 'Look! He's moving!'"

PEARLY GATES JOKES

Death, at least in the world of jokes, is usually a sterile, empty, demeaning state where there is no choice or future; this is the gray or even black world. Such are the values of our secular society. Religious outlooks often have different views about death, which may lead to entry into an afterlife, a heaven, even a New Jerusalem. Some jokes playfully uses the imagery of heaven, the Pearly Gates, and St. Peter's post at the gate. This is a liminal space, a space of transitions, much like doctors' waiting rooms, hospital lobbies, even funeral homes. If a nursing home is liminal on this side of death, St. Peter's gate is liminal immediately on the far side where, tradition says, St. Peter makes a decision about the moral status of a person's life and, therefore, the final destination, heaven or hell. St. Peter is similar to a doctor, with whom our secrets are shared and assessed, but differs in that he renders a judgment about the ultimate value of our entire life.

A joke that has resonance with the profane parrot runs like this:

Phyllis And Charlotte

In the line to St. Peter's gate a woman taps the woman ahead of her on the shoulder. "Say, aren't you Phyllis from across the street?"

"Why yes. Charlotte! Whatever are you doing here?"

"Well, I think you actually know, but I'll explain the details anyway. Regrettably, I was in bed with your husband when you came home from work early. I grabbed a sheet and thought about hiding in the bathroom, the closet, under the bed, but these were all too obvious. I ran around like a crazed person and saw the basement door. I stumbled down the steps and looked around. All I could see was the freezer, so I climbed into that, confident that this was a temporary measure. Some hours later, however, I was frozen stiff and on my way up here. And what about you?"

"Well, yes, to tell you the truth, I was getting quite suspicious of him, but I didn't know who he was seeing. When I came home that day, he was frantically trying to put on some clothes. I saw women's clothes scattered about and recognized them as yours. I was quite upset, as you can imagine, and I went looking through the house, knowing your couldn't leave without your clothes. I also thought if we could talk it out, we could work past this unfortunate event.

I looked high and low and found nothing. I even looked in the basement. I went up and confronted my husband, but he wouldn't confess to the obvious, and we had a terrible fight. I slapped him. He slugged me. When I fell, I hit my head. So here I am."

"Damn. If only you had looked in the freezer, we might both still be alive!"

In this clever joke the women haven't yet reached St. Peter's gate, so we don't know how the women will be assessed, judged, and consigned. Instead, they have a chatty visit, totally open with each other. It seems that Phyllis is not vengeful toward Charlotte for sleeping with her husband, and actually thinks they could solve the dilemma by talking it out (as opposed to her violent husband who caused her death). Oddly enough, the two women seem to have repaired their friendship in a small, comic society. Charlotte's sanguine (erotic) overdrive seems to be considered permissible in Phyllis' eyes, although not in Charlotte's, since her guilt led to her flight through the house and her death. The freezer cools her lust and gives an approximation of a casket or grave (especially in the Poe-like basement).

Here is a similar story, this time male-oriented and more elaborate. I've seen two versions; here is my retelling.

A Boring Day In Heaven

It was a boring day in heaven, because everything was perfect as usual. Saint Gabriel thought he'd stroll down to the Gate and see if Saint Peter had anything interesting to say. When he got there, however, Peter was as bored as Gabriel. They sighed and drummed their fingers on Peter's desk.

The clouds parted and a newly dead person approached the desk. Saint Peter got the name and punched it into the computer. In a second the entire record of that person flashed across the screen as well as the final judgment; in this case, the judgment was ADMITTED.

"So that's it?" asked Gabriel.

"Yeah, it's been no fun since the computer system came online. Before, I'd interview them, check the records, and make my own judgment. Now, I just poke a few keys and deliver the news."

"Pathetic," Gabriel agreed. "And I thought my job was boring."

Gabriel watched a few more candidates and thought about moving on, but he couldn't think of anywhere interesting to go.

"Say," he said.

"Yeah?"

"Look, why don't you go back to the old way. You can tell God the computer went down or the software crashed. But just for a while…why don't you ask them how they died? We'll have some interesting stories and you can make your decision based on that!"

"Wow, that's a great idea! Let's try it out." He pulled the power cord (!) out of the computer, which immediately shut down.

They watched the clouds expectantly and soon a middle-aged man appeared and came to the desk.

"How did you die?" asked Peter.

"Well, it's a strange story, but I guess I have to tell you. I came home from work early, took the elevator up to the sixth floor to my condo. I was getting out my key when I heard sounds of people in sexual ecstasy. Can't be my place, I thought, looking at the other doors, but I recognized my wife's voice. I opened the door, heard some yelling, and ran down the hall to the bedroom. There was my wife, naked and shocked to see me, and I could hear the frantic footsteps of her partner. I yelled at the man and then I chased after him. Our condo has a layout that lets you go in a circle, which I did—two or three times—but I didn't find anyone. Finally I looked through the kitchen and out onto the balcony and saw some fingers on the edge of the slab that makes the floor.

"'Aha!' I cried. I ran out and looked. Sure enough, there's some guy hanging on for dear life. 'You bastard,' I screamed. He yelled, 'No, wait!' but I'm stomping on his fingers—kind of like in "North by Northwest," when Cary Grant is holding Eve Marie Saint on Mount Rushmore—except that here it was both hands, and of course he fell—to my great satisfaction. But—get this, guys—he fell into a tree and a series of branches broke his fall so perfectly that he landed on the grass and picked himself up and started to brush himself off.

"Well, I don't mind telling you, I went berserk and grabbed the first thing I saw, the refrigerator! I ripped it out of the kitchen and heaved it over my head and hurled it over the railing at the man. It was a perfect shot. Drove him into the ground like a tent peg. Of course this adrenaline-fueled effort gave me both a stroke and a heart attack, and I collapsed on the balcony floor, and here I am."

Gabriel and Peter looked at each other with wide smiles.

"Sir, you may pass through the gate," said Peter. The man does so.

Gabriel and Peter congratulated each other on the success of this strategy, and waited expectantly.

Soon the clouds parted, and a man slightly younger than the previous one presented himself to the desk.

"How did you die?"

"Well, it's a strange story. It was such a nice day that I took my free weights out onto the balcony—I live in a condo on the seventh floor—and I was lifting in my usual routine. The space wasn't really adequate, though, and I lost my balance and fell over the railing at the edge.

"'Oh no, I'm going to die,' I thought, but I also realized that the condo below mine was built exactly the same, so I could catch the railing below. I almost accomplished this, but my hands slipped off the railing and on down until they reached the concrete slab, and here I did manage to catch myself. I was about to pull myself up when a maniac with a red face started to stomp on my fingers. 'No, wait!' I yelled, but he persisted and stomped my fingers. Of course, I had to let go and I began to fall.

"Once again I thought, 'Oh no, I'm going to die,' but I crashed through some tree branches—with some bruising, mind you—but enough to retard my fall greatly. I landed on the ground, full of joy and thanksgiving, and stood up. I was brushing myself off, when I heard a strange whistling noise overhead, and then all went black. And here I am."

Gabriel and Peter looked at each other with wide smiles.

"Sir, you may pass through the gate," said Peter. The man did so.

The two angels waited expectantly, and soon the clouds parted and another man—a young one this time—appeared. He walked up to the desk.

"How did you die?" asked Peter.

"Well, it's a strange story. Picture this: I'm hiding inside a refrigerator."

These two chiller jokes illustrate our fears of cold, narrow, grave-like places, spaces that are sterile, enclosing, and terminal. In each case, the cold is opposed to the heat of sexual lust. The joke about Charlotte and Phyllis draws on some traditional gothic imagery; we may think of Poe's "Pit and the Pendulum" or "The Cask of Amontillado," both of which use threats of burial or immurement. In the Poe stories, however, the victims are relatively innocent, in contrast to the chiller jokes, where the characters are sanguine adulterers who need a phlegmatic cooling off. Indeed death has been called "The Big Chill," as in the movie by that name (1983) in which aging Boomers gather after the death of a friend. Another image from the cinema is Jack Nicholson's crazed character in "The Shining," who is—justifiably, we feel—frozen to death. In these representations, death is final, with no promise of redemption or passage to heaven. In "Phyllis and Charlotte" the narrative stops before St. Peter's judgment, so the sanguine character remains unjudged forever.

This joke has been around for decades:

There's a long, long line at St. Peter's gate, and the newly dead grumble about the delay. Suddenly there's a commotion at the back of the line as a man in a white coat runs past people waiting. As he continues along the side of the line, it becomes clear that he's carrying a stethoscope. When he reaches the head of the line, St. Peter waves him on through. There are indignant cries of protest and outrage. St. Peter stands up at his desk and yells, "It's OK, folks. That was God Himself. Every once in a while he likes to go down there and play doctor!"

Death As A Good Thing

Most of the jokes I've seen construe death as a negative event: coffins are bad, basements are bad, freezers are bad, and St. Peter may send you to infernal perdition! Occasionally, a comic text will suggest the possibility that passing to the next world is good.

Bran Muffins

A couple had been married for sixty years. Though they were far from rich, they managed to get by because they watched their pennies. Though clearly not young, they were both in very good health, largely due to the wife's insistence on healthy foods and exercise for the last few decades.

One day, they went on a rare vacation, and their plane crashed, sending them off to Heaven. They reached the pearly gates, and St. Peter greeted them, admitted them, and escorted them inside. He took them to a beautiful mansion, furnished in gold and fine silks, with a fully stocked kitchen and a waterfall in the master bath. A maid could be seen hanging their favorite clothes in the closet. They gasped in astonishment when he said, "Welcome to Heaven. This will be your home now."

The old man asked Peter how much all this was going to cost.

Peter replied, "Why, nothing. This is your reward in Heaven."

The old man looked out the window and right there he saw a championship golf course, finer and more beautiful than any on earth.

"What are the greens fees?" grumbled the old man.

"This is heaven," St. Peter replied. "You can play for free every day."

Next they went to the clubhouse and saw the lavish buffet lunch, with every imaginable cuisine laid out before them, from seafood to steaks to exotic desserts, plus free flowing beverages.

"Don't even ask," said St. Peter to the man. "This is Heaven, it is all free for you to enjoy."

The old man looked around and glanced nervously at his wife.

"Well, where are the low-fat and low-cholesterol foods, and where's the decaffeinated tea?" he asked.

"That's the best part," St. Peter replied. "You can eat and drink as much as you like of whatever you like, and you will never get fat or sick, because this is Heaven!"

The old man pushed, "No gym to work out at?"

"Not unless you want to," was the answer.

"No testing my sugar or blood pressure or..."

"Never again. All you do here is enjoy yourself."

The old man glared at his wife and shouted: "You and your bran muffins! We could have been here ten years ago!"

Another parodist has been at work, although this one has a feeling more of play than of anger. I congratulate the anonymous author.

Heart Health Parody

Q: I've heard that cardiovascular exercise can prolong life; is this true?

A: Your heart is only good for so many beats, and that's it; don't waste them on exercise. You've got to understand that everything wears out eventually. Speeding up your heart will not make you live longer; that's like saying you can extend the life of your car by driving it faster. Want to live longer? Take a nap.

Q: Should I cut down on meat and eat more fruits and vegetables?

A: You must grasp logistical efficiencies. What does a cow eat? Hay and corn. And what are these? Vegetables. So a steak is nothing more than an efficient mechanism of delivering vegetables to your system. Need grain? Eat chicken. Beef is also a good source of field grass (a green leafy vegetable). And a pork chop can give you 100% of your recommended daily allowance of vegetable products.

Q: Should I reduce my alcohol intake?

A: No, not at all. Wine is made from fruit. Brandy is distilled wine, that means they take the water out of the fruity bit so you get even more of the goodness that way. Beer is also made out of grain. Bottoms up!

Q: How can I calculate my body/fat ratio?

A: Well, if you have a body and you have fat, your ratio is one to one. If you have two bodies, your ratio is two to one, etc.

Q: What are some of the advantages of participating in a regular exercise program?

A: Can't think of a single one, sorry. My philosophy is: No Pain...Good!

Q: Aren't fried foods bad for you?

A: YOU'RE NOT LISTENING! Foods are fried these days in vegetable oil. In fact, they're permeated in it. How could getting more vegetables be bad for you?

Q: Will sit-ups help prevent me from getting a little soft around the middle?

A: Definitely not! When you exercise a muscle, it gets bigger. You should only be doing sit-ups if you want a bigger stomach.

Q: Is chocolate bad for me?

A: Are you crazy? HELLO. Cocoa beans! Another vegetable! It's the best feel-good food around!

Q: Is swimming good for your figure?

A: If swimming is good for your figure, explain whales to me.

Q: Is getting in shape important for my lifestyle?

A: Hey! 'Round' is a shape!

Well, I hope this has cleared up any misconceptions you may have had about food and diets. And remember: "Life should NOT be a journey to the grave with the intention of arriving safely in an attractive and well preserved body, but rather to skid in sideways—Chardonnay in one hand—chocolate in the other—body thoroughly used up, totally worn out and screaming, "Whoa! What a great ride!"

Aging And Sex

In the world of humor, there's a common polarity of sex and death. Sex, as we have seen, symbolizes many aspects of health: energy, power, pleasure, freedom, and social success. Sex allows society to continue into the future as couples create children, who grow up to reproduce themselves as well; this is the Green World of fecundity and pleasure.

We're seen some jokes in this chapter and elsewhere that have a subtheme of sex as a marker of health and agency. Here are some others that emphasize aging.

Two old men are sitting on a park bench. The ninety-year-old has just finished his morning jog. The eighty-year-old admires his friend's stamina and asks him his secret.

"Rye bread. Fantastic stuff. Keeps you in the pink and you have great stamina with the ladies as well."

The younger man is intrigued. He stops by the bakery on his way home and scans the shelves.

"Can I help you?" the woman behind the counter says.

"Oh yes, I need some rye bread."

"Well, it's right here. How much?"

"I'll take five loaves."

"Gracious! Five loaves? It'll get hard."

"You mean everyone knows about rye bread except me?"

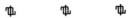

Married for thirty years, a couple gave a big party for their sixtieth birthdays. Looking down from heaven, an angel was thrilled to see this happy scene and flew down to witness the proceedings.

Later that night, as the couple was going to bed, the angel appeared privately and congratulated them, saying, "Your marriage is so exemplary, I'm going to grant you one wish."

"Great," says the wife. "I'd like two tickets for a trip around the world."

"Done," says the angel waving her wand and BINGO the wife had two tickets in her hand.

"And for you?" says the angel, turning to the husband.

"Aha. Well, quite frankly, I'd like a woman thirty years younger than me."

"Done," says the angel, waving her wand and BINGO the man is suddenly ninety years old.

The trickster is tricked, and his punishment appears correct for his sexist, churlish, and ageist behavior in rejecting his faithful wife.

Jacob, age ninety-two, and Rebecca, age eighty-nine, live in Florida, and they are all excited about their decision to get married. They go for a stroll to discuss the wedding, and on the way they pass a drugstore. Jacob suggests they go in.

Jacob addresses the man behind the counter: "Are you the owner?"

The pharmacist answers, "Yes, I am."

Jacob: "Excellent, because we have a few questions."

Pharmacist, "Fire away."

Jacob: "Well, we're about to get married. Do you sell heart medication?"

Pharmacist: "Of course we do."

Jacob: "How about medicine for circulation?"

Pharmacist: "All kinds."

Jacob: "Medicine for rheumatism and scoliosis?"

Pharmacist: "Definitely."

Jacob: "How about Viagra?"

Pharmacist: "Of course."

Jacob: "Medicine for memory problems, arthritis, jaundice?"

Pharmacist: "Yes, a large variety. The works."

Jacob: "What about vitamins, sleeping pills, Geritol, antidotes for Parkinson's disease?"

Pharmacist: "Absolutely."

Jacob: "You sell wheelchairs and walkers?"

Pharmacist: "All speeds and sizes."

Jacob: "Very well then. We'd like to use this store as our Bridal Registry."

In Summary

This chapter opened with young doctors using slang to refer to Mr. Sullivan's imminent demise but also to protect themselves from the tragedy of his death and the tragic limits of the medicine they practice. Their language is a parody of medical terms, words that sound serious to outsiders, but a code for joking among the residents. Their playful language represented their attempt to deal with aging and death. Popular culture has a wide range of jokes with parallel functions, to identify aspects of aging, loss of sexual power, and vulnerability to death, but packaging them through humorous stories that allow us a ritual of agreement that such things inevitably exist and that they are troubling but also that we can reinterpret them through humor. While we can't solve the basic dilemma of being mortal, we can, in brief comic moments, laugh at our complex relationship with aging and death.

Chapter Ten

Brunhilde Blesses the ICU

And Other Hospital Humor

WHILE I WAS working on this book, my wife and I were healthcare surrogates for a woman I had gone to college with forty-five years before. Terminally ill with cancer, she was a patient in an intensive care unit. Because the hall door was locked, we had to call on a phone by the door and state our business. Then we had to wash our hands. Then we went to the nursing station to see where our friend was. We scanned the cubicles lining the unit, each with an exterior window, each with a single, very sick patient. Unused to this strange space, we felt alienated from reality and frightened. The young doctor taking care of her was all business: scientific and rational. The nurses had more sympathy for our fear and sadness, and an unexpected bit of humor with an unknown source helped us lighten our somber emotions.

BRUNHILDE BLESSES THE ICU

Next to my friend's room was a gray cart labeled "Isolation Gowns." Visitors were required to wear these yellow paper gowns in order to guard patients against infection. One particular gown, however, was strangely taped to the top of the cabinet and cut so that it appeared to be a woman's hairdo hanging down in front of the drawers, with a set of bangs in the center and two large braids at the sides. Below the bangs were two large eyes drawn in black marker on the front of a drawer. Below them was the vertical chrome drawer handle, now converted visually to a strange, shiny nose. Below that was a large mouth (again black marker), presumably a woman's, in a wide smile.

My wife and I found this sight strange but amusing, even cheerful. It represented a playful game created by some anonymous ICU staff—although potentially any nurses or doctors we might speak with—thus suggesting other aspects of their personalities than their professional appearances. The woman's face on the cabinet, although an ersatz parody of a real person, seemed energetic and vital. I thought of this figure as the Wagnerian Brunhilde, operatic and powerful, but also comic in her own way. She provided a constant smile, a blessing of sorts, every hour of every day within the difficult confines for very sick people, a space where many caring but worried family and friends visited. Further, this artistic subversion of medical equipment told us that the healthcare workers had senses of humor much like ours, and we felt a bit more at home in an alien place. In contrast to the boisterous Party Time! humor of ER staff (and among ER staff only), Brunhilde was more of a clownish figure, gently comic and available to anyone who saw her. Blessing the unit, she could be seen as a laric figure of love.

In this chapter we'll look at humor in hospital settings or about hospitals. Some, like Brunhilde, are created by caregivers; some are created by patients; some are created by people outside hospitals.

The next exhibit, "Actual entries in hospital charts," is unusual: entries from patients' medical chart that were probably mistakes originally and certainly not jokes. The wide transmission of them via the Internet has, however, given them the status of jokes, because—disconnected from real, suffering people—they are funny. I've never seen a source for these and certainly have no idea how they might have been collected, but several versions have come to me over the past decade. If these are actual entries, many of them were probably written by exhausted physicians, especially resident doctors who had been on duty for far too many hours. Other errors may have occurred by transcriptionists working from doctors' notes read into a recorder. Whatever their sources and authenticity, these short observations have a non-sequitur nature that has apparently delighted many people. Taken as a whole, they give us pause to think about the inexactitude of language and the absurdity of the world. In the comic world, we take these as literary hypotheses, so that the implied characters are not actual, suffering people.

Actual Entries In Hospital Charts

1. Patient has chest pain if she lies on her left side for over a year.

2. On the second day the knee was better, and on the third day it disappeared.

3. The patient is tearful and crying constantly. She also appears to be depressed.

4. The patient has been depressed since she began seeing me in 1993.

5. Discharge status: alive but without my permission.

6. Healthy appearing decrepit sixty-seven-year-old male, mentally alert but forgetful.

7. The patient refused autopsy.

8. The patient has no previous history of suicides.

9. Patient has left white blood cells at another hospital.

10. Patient's medical history has been remarkably insignificant with only forty pound weight gain in the past three days.

11. Patient had waffles for breakfast and anorexia for lunch.

12. Between you and me, we ought to be able to get this lady pregnant. Since she can't get pregnant with her husband, I thought you might like to work her up.

13. She is numb from her toes down.

14. While in ER, she was examined, X-rated, and sent home.

15. The skin was moist and dry.

16. Occasional, constant infrequent headaches.

17. Patient was alert and unresponsive.

18. Rectal examination revealed a normal size thyroid.

19. She stated that she had been constipated for most of her life, until she got a divorce.

20. Both breasts are equal and reactive to light and accommodation.

21. Examination of genitalia reveals that he is circus sized.

22. The lab test indicated abnormal lover function.

23. I saw your patient today, who is still under our car for physical therapy.

24. The patient was to have a bowel resection. However, he took a job as a stockbroker instead.

25. Skin: somewhat pale but present.

26. The pelvic exam will be done later on the floor.

27. Patient was seen in consultation by Dr. XXX, who felt we should sit on the abdomen and I agree.

28. Large brown stool ambulating in the hall.

29. Patient has two teenaged children, but no other abnormalities.

30. She has no rigors or shaking chills, but her husband states she was very hot in bed last night.

The popularity of these owes greatly to several kinds of pleasure. The first is a combination of enjoying the absurd concept, while the second is figuring out what it should have been. In 21, "circus sized" gives us imaginative range, and the word probably should have been "circumcised." In 20, the animated breasts were probably, in fact, eyes. 14 and 23 are pretty clearly typos. A third source of our amusement lies in an unresolved paradox. In 8, the patient could not have a history of suicides, since s/he would already be dead. In 18, a rectal exam would not (we hope!) reach up to the throat. And, of course, we have the violation of good old taboo, as in 30, the hot woman, and 12, the docs determined to get a woman pregnant. These notes are probably funnier to persons outside the hospital and in relatively good health. To be in a hospital where mistakes might have dire consequences would be troubling.

Another exhibit, "Actual comments made during colonoscopies," is similarly anonymous. This came as an email with the explanation that a physician had collected them while treating patients, most of whom were male.

> Actual Comments During Colonoscopies
> 1. Take it easy, Doc. You're boldly going where no man has gone before!
> 2. Find Amelia Earhart yet?
> 3. Can you hear me NOW?'
> 4. Are we there yet? Are we there yet? Are we there yet?
> 5. You know, in Arkansas, we're now legally married.
> 6. Any sign of the trapped miners, Chief?
> 7. You put your left hand in, you take your left hand out....
> 8. Hey! Now I know how a Muppet feels!
> 9. If your hand doesn't fit, you must quit!
> 10. Hey Doc, let me know if you find my dignity.
> 11. You used to be an executive at Enron, didn't you?
> 12. God, now I know why I am not gay.
> 13. Could you write a note for my wife saying that my head is not up there?

Similar to the humor about mammograms we saw earlier, these are attempts by the patients to gain some emotional control over a stressful situation. Number 10 is the most direct in identifying a loss of dignity, as if such could be hidden in the bowel. Despite the differences in these, they all show the turmoil of patients subjected to anal penetration. Several of them refer to fear of being gay.

Another exhibit satirizes medical terms in alphabetical order; it has circulated for years under a variety of titles. At least four nurses have given it to me. Why do they like it? Nurses are under constant pressure to administer the right medicines, to chart exactly, and to speak accurately to patients and their families. Many nurses are women, and women often like verbal play. Perhaps most important is a claim for freedom by redefining medical terms in terms of life outside the hospital.

The entries are all puns (of varying degrees of wit) purporting to redefine medical terms in a wider cultural context. I've combined several versions.

Hospital Terminology

Artery	the study of paintings
Bacteria	the back door to the cafeteria
Barium	what doctors do when patients die
Bowel	a letter like a, e, i, o , or u
Cesarean Section	a neighborhood in Rome
Cat Scan	searching for kitty
Cauterize	made eye contact with her
Colic	a kind of sheep dog
Coma	a punctuation mark
Congenital	friendly
Dilate	to live long
Enema	not a friend
Enteritis	a penchant for burglary
Fibrillate	to tell lies
G.I. series	baseball game between soldiers
ICU	peek-a-boo
Impotent	distinguished, well known
Medical staff	a doctor's cane
Minor operation	coal digging
Morbid	a higher offer
Nitrate	cheaper than the day rate
Node	was made aware of
Outpatient	patient who fainted
Pap smear	paternity allegation
Protein	in favor of teenagers
Post-operative	a letter carrier
Recovery room	a place to do upholstery
Rectum	damn near killed 'em
Serology	a study of English knighthood
Terminal illness	getting sick at the airport
Tumor	an extra pair
Urine	opposite of you're out
Varicose	nearby
Vein	conceited

(I've not seen a version which attempts the letters w, x, y, or z.)

One version of this list was printed up by a medical office as "Medical Terminology for the Layman." Other versions suggest stupidity on the part of lay persons, as in the "Blonde Dictionary of Medical Terms" and even "Bill Clinton's Medical Dictionary," perhaps suggesting that Southerners (or hicks in general) are dumb and speak in dialect ("node" for "knowed" and "impotent" for "important"). While these are one-shot jokes with none of the resources of a narrative to deepen them, their popularity suggests a need to translate such terms out of the one-dimensional medical realm and into a realm of playful foolishness where we have some control and the right to whimsical redefinition. Some versions of this alphabet have been posted on staff bulletin boards in hospitals. As such, they are forms of play, attempts at levity in a subculture where all of the terms have serious, even life-and-death meanings. "Terminal illness" is perhaps the most obvious example of a softening of meaning, a euphemism by means of a pun.

OTHER INSTANCES

In a cubicle at a large academic hospital where a support person labored, I saw a framed plaque printed up as if it were embroidered:

> THIS JOB IS A TEST,
> AND ONLY A TEST.
> IF IT WERE A REAL JOB,
> YOU'D HAVE BONUSES,
> RAISES, AND PROMOTIONS.

Listeners to radio will recognize the format of a public service announcement for an emergency network revised here for a satiric purpose. Anyone who has had a low-level job will recognize the sentiments expressed, a direct Freudian attack on bureaucracy that does not reward support personnel, although casting the second sentence in the second person, "you," allows any viewer of the plaque to feel demeaned and perhaps also rebellious. Evidently administrators who saw it on the wall decided not to make an issue of it, because I saw it displayed over the course of a year.

AT THE POISON CENTER

I was observing at a poison center many years ago, where calls from distressed citizens were answered by well trained staff. I was given a partially disabled headset so that I could hear these conversations but not make any utterance or cough (or chuckle) that could be heard. Since calls came in sporadically, with no set pattern, I had plenty of time to interview the counselors and to scan the shelves in front of us where many reference works were readily available. I saw notebooks with CYTT handwritten on the spines. These initials stood for "Can You Top This?" Counselors wrote up the wackiest, craziest, and/or most ignorant inquiries the center received over the years, for example, "How long should the rinse cycle be for a turkey I'm washing in the washing machine?" While the counselors had the duty to treat every call seriously and politely, they took a form of revenge by recording the looniest ones so that all workers could laugh at the anonymous callers and, by extension, some of the stupidity of human beings. Here are a few more calls.

"The dog ate a box of sanitary napkins; what should we do?"

"My son swallowed a battery for a watch. How long before it runs out?"

"I enjoy belching. Can you recommend some foods for me to eat?"

"We served dinner early to our children so that dinner guests could eat later, you know, quietly. The children are now vomiting. What should we tell our guests?"

Medical Training

The rigor and tedium of medical school is often relieved by jokes, from dirty mnemonics to student follies (some of which parody professors), from practical jokes (irradiating a film badge so that the owner will get a call from the safety committee) to "wake-up" slides (professors put an incongruous slide in the middle of a lecture). One attending physician encouraged her residents to write limericks about surgical patients as a way to laugh together and blow off steam. In *First Cut*, I reported a joke about medical hierarchies (p. 164). In shortened form, it goes like this:

Sex: Work Or Play?

Big Doctor is on rounds with residents and medical students. They visit a woman recovering from hip surgery; she asks if she can resume sexual relations. Big Doctor says, "Well, if sex were play, I'd say yes, but since we all know it's work, I'll have to give the order no." The chief resident agrees heartily. A first-year resident, hoping for brownie points, cites a journal article to that effect. A fourth-year medical student, also hustling, does likewise. When Big Doctor asks (pimps, in medical slang) a first-year student for his opinion, he says, "Actually, it's 100 per cent play."

"What," cries Big Doctor, "Your proof? Statistics?"

"Naaaa. I just know that if there was any work involved, I'd be doing yours."

This joke was offered in an anatomy lecture by a professor. The first-year students laughed uproariously, well aware of their low positions and the scut work they'd be soon be doing for everyone senior to them. Besides a rebellious edge to the humor, there is also the criticism that the workloads for medical students (not to mention residents) are often unreasonable. Satire in medical student follies is often a combination of silliness for silliness' sake as well as satirical comment. Barron H. Lerner writes that such follies often have serious aims to improve medical education but that some of the wilder humor has been tempered, now that there are more women students. He also notes that the advent of YouTube has greatly increased access to material that was formerly private, in-house, backstage, and in a limited comic community.[1] No doubt an entire book could be devoted to describing and interpreting humor and medical training; Suzanne Poirier's *Doctors in the Making* analyzes many student memoirs and mentions gallows humor (p. 117), but most topics raised in her study are serious.[2]

INTERSERVICE RIVALRIES

Since the Renaissance, the barber-surgeons and the physicians have represented two different strands of medical practice. (Even today's title the "Columbia College of Physicians and Surgeons" reflects this division.) The folklore of medical humor has this formulation:

> Internal medicine doctors know everything and do nothing.
>
> Surgeons know nothing and do everything.
>
> Pathologists know everything and do everything—but a day late.

While we chuckle at the indirect reference to death, the joke embodies our fears that medicine is indeed limited, even while we hope that it can do everything to keep us healthy and happy forever. Nor do we like the notion that some knowledge is useless, as in the following, a joke cheerfully told to me by a pediatrician.

Holmes And Watson Go Ballooning

Sherlock Holmes and Dr. Watson are stumped on a particularly difficult case. Sherlock ponders and ponders and announces, "Watson! I have it! We must hire a balloon straightaway! And bring your service revolver!"

"Very good, Holmes."

They hire a balloon, climb into the basket, and rise above London.

"Aha," cries Holmes, surveying the rooftops, "This shall certainly provide the information we require!"

"Most excellent," says Dr. Watson.

As they drift along, however, a thick fog advances toward them, obscuring the Tower Bridge, St. Paul's, and the Houses of Parliament, although they can still hear Big Ben.

"Damn and blast," cries Holmes. "We must lower to orient ourselves."

They descend and miraculously a hole in the fog allows them to see a man seated on a park bench. But which park?

"Hallooo, I say, halloo!" calls out Holmes. "Just where might we be located?"

The man puts down his newspaper and looks up.

"Well now, sir," the man returns. "I should say you were one hundred forty-three feet from me at a seventy-seven degree angle."

"Yes, but....," Holmes starts; however, the fog closes in and an updraft carries the balloon suddenly away.

"How do you like that," says Dr. Watson. "Of all the people we might question, we hit upon a neurologist."

"A neurologist?" asks Holmes (usually the one, of course, to make bold, deductive leaps).

"Obviously," replies Dr. Watson. "He gave us perfectly accurate information that is completely useless."

Neurology is one of the stranger areas for medical research, because the human brain is so complex and mysterious. Other physicians sometimes take a satiric poke at neurologists, whose work seems to epitomize the unsolved problems that face all specialists.

A more elaborate joke satirizes not one but five specialties, still with the theme that each of them has inherent limitations. I first heard this joke at a medical school in 1983; other versions have circulated since then.

Doctors Go Duck Hunting

Five physicians—an internist, a pediatrician, a psychiatrist, a surgeon, and a pathologist—went duck hunting together. They agreed that when ducks came overhead, they should not all shoot together, because they wouldn't know who should get credit for any kills. The surgeon insisted that he should be first, but the psychiatrist successfully counseled them to draw straws and shoot in the prescribed order. This done, they lined up in the hunting blind. The surgeon was singularly unhappy, because he was to go next to last.

The internist was the first to take aim at a flock of ducks flying overhead. However, as he raised his gun, certain decision trees and calculations filled his mind: "60% likelihood that these are ducks, but 20% possibility of teal, and at least 12% widgeons or other waterfowl; perhaps a second opinion would be indicated." Of course, by this time, the ducks were safely out of range.

The pediatrician now took his turn as the second flock appeared. However, he too was beset by doubt: "Perhaps there are mother ducks here; perhaps they had babies; some may be too young and/or have developmental issues." As he warred with himself, the ducks flew safely away.

Another flock soon followed and the psychiatrist took aim. As he viewed the ducks, he questioned: "Yes, they are ducks to my perceptions; but is, in fact, their self-image truly duck-like? Deep down, do they know they are ducks?" As he pondered this dilemma, the ducks flew safely out of harm's way.

The next group of birds flew overhead. The surgeon swiftly took aim and, without hesitation, fired multiple times. His shots were accurate, and many birds fell out of the sky. The surgeon turned to the pathologist and said: "Go out and see whether any of those were ducks!"

Another version concludes: The surgeon elbows the other doctors aside initially then shoots every bird out of the sky for two miles around. He swats the dog on the behind and yells, "Get out there so we can see what we got!" Perri Klass has another version that pokes fun at an ER physician in her *Not an Entirely Benign Procedure*.[3]

In the following joke, the rivals are all microsurgeons. Satire treats competitiveness, advanced medical technologies, and employment issues.

Following their professional conference in the Bahamas, several microsurgeons were getting drunk on a patio overlooking the ocean. The vista before them was impressive and large, much like their egos.

The first, from England, bragged, "One of my more interesting cases involved a man who had a most regrettable industrial accident. All the paramedics could recover was his little finger. Luckily, my team was ready to go and we built a hand, an arm, and the rest of the body. Indeed he went back to work and worked so well that he replaced five other people who are now out of work."

"Oh that's nothing," the American said, "We had a worker who got stuck in a nuclear reactor, leaving nothing but his hair. Using DNA analysis and some very fancy techniques that you surely don't have yet, we built him from the top down. He is now so efficient that he's replaced 40 people who are now out of work."

"Piffle, said a surgeon from [name your country!]. "As I was walking down the street one day, I smelled a fart. Luckily I had a rubber glove in my briefcase, so I captured it and brought it to the Operating Room. My team is so good that we could build the asshole, the entire ass, and the rest of the body. The resulting man is now [name the governmental official!] who is putting the entire country out of work."

We've seen humor regarding signs for doctors in Chapter Five. Here is a more extended version that pits medical arts versus social taboos:

Dr. Smith And Dr. Jones

Two doctors opened an office in a small town and put up a sign reading: "Dr. Smith and Dr. Jones, Psychiatry and Proctology."

The town council was unhappy with that sign because it suggested local citizens were crazy and/or had unmentionable problems, so the doctors changed it to "Hysterias and Posteriors." This was not acceptable either, so in an effort to satisfy the council, they changed the sign to "Schizoids and Hemorrhoids." Still no go!

Next they tried "Catatonics and High Colonics." Thumbs down again.

Then came, "Manic-depressives and Anal-retentives." Still not good.

How about, "Minds and Behinds"? Unacceptable again.

So they tried, "Lost Souls and Ass Holes." No good.

Neither did "Analysis and Anal Cysts," "Nuts and Butts," "Freaks and Cheeks," nor "Loons and Moons" have any success.

Almost at their wits' end, the doctors finally came up with a title they thought might be acceptable to the council: "Dr. Smith and Dr. Jones, Odds and Ends."

Besides the play with words and taboos, we have a dual focus on mental acuity and anality, suggesting that we are deeply concerned with our mental health and the health of our bowels. The two doctors work at the top and the bottom of the spine, our central mast. (In Hindu tradition, the chakras line up on the spine from the anus to the top of the head.) An underlying sense of the joke is this: what does it mean to be human and how many things can go wrong with our brains (our sanity) and our bowels (one of our most basic organs)? In our society, mental illness is often taboo as well as references to the anus, bowels, and feces.

SATIRE AND PARODY

Satire makes fun of a person, an institution, even an idea. In the following, the speaker could be called either phlegmatic or stupid, while the notion of self-help gets satiric treatment as well.

Self Help

I have found inner peace, yes, true inner peace.

The breakthrough came at 3:00 a.m., when I couldn't sleep and turned on my television. There a man with a real doctor's degree was telling how you could find inner peace. He said that you should not have unfinished business in your life. He said you should finish stuff that you started.

So I gave my life some careful thought and looked around the house.

I finished off a bottle of chardonnay, a bottle of Grand Marnier, some Bristol Crème, two boxes of cookies, a box of raisins, some frozen take-home packages from restaurants, and a just-started box of chocolates.

Sleep came easy after that because I had gained true and lasting inner peace.

Here's another Biblical-sounding (like Eve's three breasts in Chapter Six) piece that satirizes unhealthy fashions in food. This came as a forwarded email; I congratulate the original, anonymous author for the social criticism it offers.

God's Diet

In the beginning God covered the earth with broccoli, cauliflower, and spinach, green, yellow, and red vegetables of all kinds; so Man and Woman would live long and healthy lives. And God created the healthful yogurt that Woman might keep the figure that Man found so fair.

But Satan created Ben and Jerry's and Krispy Kreme. And Satan said, "You want hot fudge with that?" And Man said, "Yes!" and Woman said, "I'll have another with sprinkles!" And lo, they gained 10 pounds.

And Satan brought forth white flour from the wheat, and sugar from the cane, and high-fructose corn syrup. And Woman went from size 2 to size 10.

So God said, "Try my fresh green salad." But Satan presented crumbled Bleu Cheese dressing and garlic toast on the side.

And Man and Woman unfastened their belts following the repast.

God then said, "I have sent you heart healthy vegetables and olive oil in which to cook them."

But Satan brought forth deep-fried coconut shrimp, butter-dipped lobster chunks and chicken-fried steak so big it needed its own platter. And Man's cholesterol went through the roof.

God then brought forth running shoes so that his Children might lose those extra pounds.

And Satan came forth with a cable TV with remote control so Man would not have to toil changing the channels. And man and woman laughed and cried before the flickering light and started wearing stretch jogging suits.

Then God brought forth the potato, naturally low in fat and brimming with potassium and good nutrition. Then Satan peeled off the healthful skin and sliced the starchy center into chips and deep-fried them in animal fats and added copious quantities of salt. And Man put on more pounds.

God then gave lean beef so that Man might consume fewer calories and still satisfy his appetite. And Satan created McDonald's and the 99-cent double cheeseburger. Then Lucifer said, "You want fries with that?" and Man replied, "Yes! And super size' em!" And Satan said, "It is good." And Man went into cardiac arrest.

God sighed and created quadruple bypass surgery.

And Satan created HMOs.

Amen.

In Summary

From Brunhilde to God's Diet, we have a wide variety of ways healthcare personnel, patients, and lay people use humor to change the emotions and meanings involved with medical subjects. Some jokes, like "Sex: Work or Play?" display Freudian attack, while "Dr. Smith and Dr. Jones" are largely for the fun of the wordplay and toying with taboos but with no deeper meanings.

Chapter Eleven

Rabid Fluffy, the Emergency Room Scapedog

WHEN I CAME for my Wednesday afternoons in the ER, I would sign in with the Chaplain's Office and the Volunteers' Office, put on my red volunteer's jacket, and push through the double doors that read:

NO ADMITTANCE
ER STAFF ONLY

I'd tell the unit clerk and the charge nurse that I had arrived, wash my hands, and look around the unit to see who was available to visit. While there was always variation in the patients and their disasters, the routine of the ER was fairly stable and predictable. Doctors and nurses attended to patients, wrote in charts, exchanged information, talked to relatives, and so on.

Over one period of about six weeks, however, there was an unusual development: a running joke about Fluffy. I never learned who originated the joke, but I found the source of the image: a publication called *Rabies Concepts for Medical Professionals*. This was an inexpensively produced, large-format booklet that had on its cover a black and white photograph of the head of a German Shepherd with its mouth open, teeth bared, and much saliva dripping. This disquieting image—roughly life-sized—filled most of the cover, with the title below. Our ER bookshelves held phone books and references of all sorts, from expensive medical textbooks to more ephemeral material such as this rabies text. Ordinarily the rabies booklet sat there unused and ignored, but perhaps in a rare moment of inactivity, maybe after midnight, a nurse had seen the rabies booklet, said "Aha!" and taken it to the copy machine.

Over several weeks, images of this threatening dog appeared in a variety of strange and imaginative forms. Fluffy's head was shrunk down and superimposed onto news photos and advertisements and posted on bulletin boards, taped to file cabinets, and placed where other nurses would see these folkloric creations. One full-sized photo was enhanced with highlighter so that the eyes were an arresting pink and the open, drooling mouth a brilliant yellow; this was placed on a file cabinet where everyone could see it.

Another image, which was called "Snowball," was a photo of an even more clearly vicious dog—a bulldog with ears and dogtags flying—dramatically challenging the photographer. His mouth was open, teeth bared, eyes slitted. Behind his head a double chain led from his heavy leather collar back to his handler, whose fist gripped the chain. We saw parts of human legs braced against the dog's lunge, but that was all; the faceless handler was shadowy, generic. This photograph was a portion of a newspaper or magazine spread, but not enough to identify further. Like Fluffy, Snowball was thematically scary, although it had the intensification of willed aggression: I assume this was a trained attack dog, a weapon of power of the shadowy handler and his world—especially troubling after the events at Abu Ghraib in Iraq.

On the other hand, the German Shepherd, Fluffy, could be a family pet that contracted a mortal and dangerous disease that can be randomly and violently spread to humans "in the wrong place at the wrong time." While Snowball's threat of violence was well defined and (we hope) strictly managed, Fluffy's rabid threat of violence and disease was more chaotic and absurd, more generally possible at any time in the society at large.

Both photos were designed to use a shocking image to grab our attention, aiming the dogs straight at us with unfriendly faces and teeth bared. In each case, the graphic artist and the editor wanted to startle us but also confront us with something like: "this is part of reality, folks—deal with it," even though the two intended audiences differed: the photo that became Fluffy was aimed to a medical audience, while the other that became Snowball was in a newspaper for a general audience. But both are kin in violence and threat, symbolizing a world of danger—danger that exists in medical settings but also in society in general, and both appealed to jokers in the Emergency Room.

I never learned how the names "Fluffy" and "Snowball" originated. Clearly, they represent values that are ironic, given the images of ferocious dogs. Such names suggest fur that is clean, brushed, and white. These are names for puppies, kittens, chicks, and ducklings, all small and harmless, all domesticated and tame.

Since I also had access to the copy machine, I made copies of as many of these as I could find on Wednesdays and put them in a folder. I have thirty-four exhibits, including the two original images of ferocious dogs, fifteen modified news stories, six modified ads, four cartoons, one parody of an internal hospital campaign, and five that I'll call "free," since they're hard to classify. Many of these were posted in the nurses' lounge, but some were posted out in the charting area where nurses, doctors, technicians, the unit clerk, and volunteers could see them or even contribute. Some were visible to patients and families—more about this later.

Many people spend a large portion of their lives in offices. Often there is boredom and lethargy. Sometimes, to combat the tedium and the relentless sameness, people exchange jokes when they meet, on the phone, or on email. Sometimes there are comic postings on bulletin boards or in bathroom stalls. Such behavior has the symbolic meaning of play, creativity, and freedom; it is a form of "soft rebellion," using office resources and company time for non-related, recreational purposes. The images and stories of Fluffy (and later Snowball) in the ER richly partake of the tradition of office humor.

News Stories And Photos

ER nurses enjoyed posting strange news stories that demonstrated that the world was indeed a bizarre place. One clipping had the headline, "TWO MEN BATTLE OVER PARKING SPACE." This brief story reported that two elderly men were duking it out over a parking space. It concluded with the irony that the space was, in fact, reserved for handicapped drivers—which neither of the men were. It seemed to me that ER personnel enjoyed external confirmation that the world was routinely a bizarre and unsettled place, so that the many strange accidents that befell our patients were, in some sense, normal, and ER workers were normal in being able to laugh at—and thereby reject—oddities of every sort.

Whether in print or electronic forms, news stories are commonplace, formalized and simplified gossip about our world. Although labeled "news," such stories are often a form of entertainment that is highly conventional and predictable. They provide structures and topics that are readily subverted by jokers, as in *News of the Weird*, the Darwin Awards discussed earlier, or "The Daily Show" on TV, all featuring the unexpected, the bizarre, and the absurd—to the delight of a large number of readers and viewers who may feel comforted that their trials are, by contrast, minimal.

As the Fluffy theme evolved, news stories and photos had two kinds of modification by ER personnel, graphic and textual. One photo showed a dog receiving a rabies shot, with Fluffy's ferocious head superimposed on the body of a cuddly puppy. In another, a baseball player delivering a pitch had Fluffy's head beneath his baseball cap. Another showed a cheesecake swimsuit model with her two dogs, which sported the disproportionately large heads of Fluffy and Snowball; the caption was been modified to use the name of an actual ER employee with "her two Great *Lovers*" (instead of "Great Danes").

The front page of *Parade* magazine (an epitome of middle class propriety) featured the story "Should You Buy That Doggie in the Window?" upon which Snowball's ferocious face was superimposed. Another doctored photo showed a man dragging a child back from the ocean, from which Fluffy's head emerged, as if it were a shark or some other threatening monster. In a photo of youths playing soccer, Fluffy's head was substituted for the ball, as several boys kicked at him—a rare reversal of power relationships. Was the maker of this image expressing a wish to control the chaos that came to the ER?

The changes in accompanying text were more sophisticated and often more elaborate. A news photo of a steeplejack worker atop a tower was swinging a sledgehammer while an added Fluffy climbed toward him from below; there were two versions of this photo, with two different interpretations, one negative, the other positive —a game within the game. The first added text identified the man as a current ER nurse pursued by the ferocious Fluffy, while the second explained that a friendly Fluffy wanted to *fetch* the sledgehammer.

A last example: a news story described how a 97-pound German Shepherd/Labrador mix was hit by a car and thrown 39 feet and into a man's head. The dog was injured and taken to the ER in our hospital (the name typed in to hide the actual veterinary clinic). Below in large letters was added: FLUFFY STRIKES AGAIN! (If there was news about the man, it was apparently trimmed off.)

Advertisements

Print ads seek to catch our attention and influence our behavior; indeed the very word "advertisement" has, we may recall, Latin roots meaning "turn toward," as if our heads are turned toward an advertised product. The urge to parody or sub-vert (with roots meaning "turn under") came out clearly in the Fluffy-enhanced ads. Most of these are playful and light, but some are somewhat darker in mood.

A Metropolitan Museum of Art advertisement for an elaborate statuette of Cinderella had Fluffy's head carefully inserted onto the photo, and the title altered to "Cinderfluffy."

Pictures of Fluffy and Snowball were placed in careful symmetry on a full-page prophylactics ad with the original text "DOCTOR, WHICH CONDOM SHOULD WE USE?"

A hand-written page proclaimed a Fluffy fan club, offering a glossy photo, a set of Fluffy dog tags, and a free series of rabies shots. Requests were to be mailed to one of the regular ER physicians. This pretend ad was not a graphic or textual subversion of a photocopied document, but a parody created from scratch, with, of course, the standard picture of Fluffy.

A more ambiguous mood surrounded a large ad for the movie *Jaws: The Revenge*, with a picture of Fluffy superimposed.

For me, the saddest of the lot was a version of an appeal for missing and exploited children. "Have you seen me?" with data (age, weight, hair, eyes, etc.) for Fluffy. Here we find the poignancy of kidnapped and abused children (some of whom came to our ER) and perhaps a subtler point—since the word "puppies" replaces "children"—that the rabid and vicious Fluffy was once a pet in some family's home, once an *innocent* (in the literal meaning of "not harming").

A Hospital Promotion
Hospital administrators love internal programs intended to boost the morale of the staff. I've seen several, and each time I've heard staffers make fun of such programs and the expense it must have cost. In my ER, a large picture of Fluffy was accompanied by congratulatory text proclaiming that Fluffy had won a First Prize for Excellence in a campaign that was currently underway, all carefully prepared on an   11 x 14 poster to mimic actual awards displayed elsewhere.

Other Exhibits
Snowball and Fluffy were also transformed into masks: large photos of each (Snowball wearing a pilot's cap and goggles) were pasted on to tongue depressors as handles, and the eyes were carefully cut out. What might it mean if we held such a mask to our face and looked out? Do we contain elements of potential violence and harm that we keep suppressed within ourselves?

Another photo shows four washing machines at a Laundromat; a man is leaning into one machine, his head not visible. An arrow identifies him as a current ER doctor, while printing over his head asks, "Fluffy, where are you?" Over two neighboring machines float the images of Fluffy and Snowball. There's no evidence that they've been cleansed in any way.

Cartoons
The corpus of Fluffy and Snowball exhibits is completed by four published and photocopied cartoons picturing canines. These are interesting both as professional art intended to amuse viewers and because three of them actually have the word "Fluffy" in the original drawing. The first cartoon (without "Fluffy" originally in it) shows a grinning caricature of a dog looking at a fire hydrant with a "Wet Paint" sign; the dog has an added thought balloon that reads "I think I will." "Fluffy" is written on the side of the dog, presumably by an ER hand. Perhaps Fluffy reads "Wet Paint" as Verb Noun, not Adjective Noun. The remaining three name Fluffy in their original printing; two have male-female themes.

The first, which appeared in *The New Yorker*, shows a C. Barsotti canine on the phone asking the information operator for Fluffy, in Larchmont. (I know this origin because I cut it out and brought it in: my sole contribution to the proceedings.) It had no modifications. The last two cartoons have small dogs in living rooms; ER hands have superimposed Fluffy heads on them. In each case, the dog and a cat have made shambles of the place. In one (I believe it is signed Ev Cheney), a parrot explains to a woman at the door, groceries in her arms, "It all started when Fluffy tried to eat out of Scooter's dish." Furniture is upset and damaged, curtains hang awry, even plaster on the wall is cracked. Fluffy has been an agent of chaos. In the second (I believe signed by Tony Rose), there is similar damage, but the mood is festive. There is food and drink by the couch facing the television, one bowl labeled "FLUFFY." There's also an open box labeled "cat food," presumably provided by the thoughtful host. Fluffy is seeing the cat out the front door, and the caption is "I had a great time too!" Here Fluffy is again an agent of destruction, but the cartoon can be interpreted as depicting the end of a hot date, canine male energy and feline female energy having torn up the place. It's unclear which creature is speaking, but the "too" makes clear that the feeling is mutual.

These cartoons suggest the complex dynamics of male-female interaction, yearning, fighting, or making love. The symbolism through animals suggests the basic worlds of violence and sex that are important to humans, who, nonetheless often hide or mask them with taboos.

INTERPRETING FLUFFY AND SNOWBALL

What are we to make of these strange images and the motivations of their creators? I leaf through the folder with amusement, mild disgust, some outright laughter. I think about motivations of the people who played the Fluffy/Snowball game. Themes we have been working so far are readily apparent.

NAMING PAST TABOO

The very name "Fluffy" is ironic, sarcastic, gloriously absurd in the polarity between niceness and evil: giving that name to this dog emphasizes this disparity. There's also the ambiguity of whether it's a boast that chaos can be domesticated through this naming, or whether there's despair that the distance is too far to close, thus a sardonic recognition of danger beyond our control. In either case, the evil and absurdity are named, symbolized, and recognized as existing in our world. Comic language, even in its exaggerations, can be an honest pointer to reality. Sometimes it's the equivalent of the little child who pointed at the Emperor and cried out that he wore no clothes.

Ordinarily we consider a large rabid dog as a terrible threat, and we often deal with it by not mentioning it: it is taboo. In the ER however, examples of chaos, evil, and absurdity are routinely wheeled in the door day and night, but especially on Friday and Saturday night, when people, drink, drive, and fight.

The photographic images of Fluffy don't "name past taboo" using words per se, but they similarly use images to break taboo and to domesticate the implied threats. Shrinking the images of Fluffy and Snowball and putting them inside Cinderella's clothes or a pilot's cap and goggles suggests limitation and control of the canine threats. These are not absolute controls, more like playful strategies or hopeful hypotheses: *what if a rabid dog could be transformed into a polite princess in a lovely gown?*

Naming is a first step in recognizing unpleasant material, but the adventures of Fluffy and Snowball clearly go beyond that. As their images and names were combined with news stories, advertisements, and cartoons, they entered a dialectic with known or standard forms of publication—messages we routinely see in this culture. This dialectic is, however, ambiguous: are the dogs domesticated by their insertion into safe formats, or do they disrupt and destroy their new homes? This dilemma need not be resolved: esthetic forms, whether paintings or poems, may give us pleasure as we reflect on multiple meanings, or even no meanings at all. Perhaps the underlying meaning is as simple as this: Fluffy (evil) can be named and controlled by humorous play. If this is true, we need not fear evil as a threat.

The masks of Fluffy and Snowball particularly interest me, since they suggest a relationship between the images of vicious dogs and humans. First, there's the implied joker, who holds the mask up to his face; he tries on this projection of part of himself, the angry, snarling, combative animal that society has made him tame and hide. It's a hypothetical face that expresses anger and rage, probably related to cumulative stress. Second, and more speculatively, the wearer of these masks could be anyone, any of us. We all have Jekyll and Hyde characteristics.

IMAGERY

In the Fluffy materials, both the masks and the photographic images played a central role. Like verbal symbols, these are representations that can be manipulated in many ways, depending on the wit and craftsmanship of the person—the joker— with scissors, copy machine, marker, Scotch tape, etc.

From time to time we see the following phrase in medicine: "medicine with a human face," suggesting the ideal that medicine should not only be technical and scientific; it's a phrase for conferences and essays. (We never see "medicine with the crazed face of an animal," except in popular culture media, such as horror movies.) The Fluffy exhibits were posted to be seen and often used graphic forms that could be seen from a distance. They parallel one aspect of the professional life in the ER: the visual assessment of patients, X-rays, and printed information, but in a whimsical way that can range from Cinderella to Jaws.

Fluffy and Snowball are clearly images of danger from the animal world, subversions or perversions of "man's best friend." In the ER game, their heads are now mobile and malleable: they can appear almost anywhere, evoking the world of emergencies, tragic events that emerge from the ordinary, safe events of daily life. When a man comes in with a chainsaw injury, it's a dramatic injury for the staff to see, assess, and treat, and a tremendous change in the life of the injured man. A tool betrays its user, and dogs (typically domestic pets) can similarly become dangerous. Their animal heritage gives them the speed, strength, and sharp teeth to attack and injure an unarmed human. Because they can quickly close the distance between us and them and inflict harm to our bodies, they provide a gothic image of entrapment, enclosure, unavoidable attack and consequent pain, domination, even disfigurement.

More specifically, we fear images of aggressive, fully fanged jaws, yet we put them into stories. We think of the fascination of audiences by the movie *Jaws* and the sequel; indeed *Jaws II* was one of the transformations of Fluffy. Whether it's a nature program with a very brief image of a large animal catching prey and biting its head or neck to kill it, or the human character "Jaws" with metal teeth in a James Bond movie, we marvel at the direct intimacy of a powerful mouth destroying a living creature. When our own mouths rip flesh from bone at the dinner table, we feel power and immediate satisfaction. These notions appear in Greek tragedy as *sparagmos*, or the ripping apart of a person as in *The Bacchae* or in the recent movies of *Braveheart* and *The Passion of Christ*—both Mel Gibson efforts. These are not comedies, of course, but other representations of evil and violence that may threaten us. TV fare about hospitals and clinics commonly uses the formula of mixing tragedy, comedy, and melodrama from *M*A*S*H* to *St. Elsewhere*, from *Chicago Hope* to *ER*, *Crossing Jordan*, and *House*.

Even the severed heads of the two dogs are richly ambiguous. Are they free-floating "biting heads" that can surprise us at any moment? Or are they decapitated and therefore nonthreatening?

CHARACTER

The images of the dogs are quicksilver in the hands of the ER jokers, available for a wide range of characteristics: as ferocious and dangerous as Nemesis, or as silly and tame as Cinderella with a dog's head. Either way, they have no depth, no ability to change; they are fixed ciphers that the jokers can control by photocopied size and whimsical placement. These activities suggest the jokers' domestication and control of evil and chaos; indeed the entire game taken as a whole suggests an allegory for the work of the ER in general: facing and rectifying all absurdities that patients bring.

While Fluffy and Snowball are arresting characters, perhaps the most interesting characters are actually the anonymous jokers of the ER who manipulated these images and who, day after day, steadfastly meet the needs of patients in the ER.

STORY

When I asked nurses, "What's the deal with Fluffly?" I learned that there were two framing stories. The first was that Fluffy had entered the ER, bit several persons, then disappeared upstairs, presumably causing trouble in the medical floors above us. This basic narrative parallels the journey of a patient who is seen and treated in the ER then admitted and sent upstairs for further treatment. One interpretation could be that Fluffy, symbolizing danger and chaos ("biting several people") passed through the ER, which did its job, and then the next group of medical personnel took up the task. We can see this as a variation on the Night Sea Journey: the ER personnel stay fixed but the underworld comes to them, stays a while, then moves on to challenge other doctors and nurses.

The second story that emerged is shorter and terminal. One Wednesday I came to the ER for my shift and looked around for the latest Fluffy and Snowball folklore. Not only was there nothing new, there was nothing at all anywhere. When I could find a moment with a nurse who had been one of the players, I asked him, "Hey, what happened to Fluffy?"

"Oh, he died."

"Really! Did someone kill him?"

"Damn straight—the hospital administration. They figured some of the patients could see some of our stuff, and that was the end of it."

He needed to say no more. I had worked in offices where bulletin board humor had gotten out of hand and bosses had reined in the activity. The nurse who informed me felt some resentment about the end of the game, but he also accepted it because he knew the reason made sense: patients, visitors, or family members could see some of the images. They could not be considered part of the comic community; indeed they might be horrified by some of the postings.

We can interpret Fluffy through the tradition of the scapegoat. By a mythic reading, Fluffy carries away the values of evil, absurdity, and chaos of the ER to the floors upstairs. As common workplace expressions put it, "it's their problem now" and "off my desk and on to theirs." In the second story of Fluffy's death by the administration, he carries the bad values into the grave. Our society seems to find satisfaction in having scapegoats taking the blame or the fall, even if other persons are equally or more at fault. Scapegoating is as American as apple pie, and gives us feelings of justice and finality.

What did the Fluffy and Snowball game mean for the nurses and physicians? The employees are long dispersed; I can't interview them. (And I'm not sure they'd know what it meant; I think they acted without much thought to deeper meanings.) The Fluffy players used canine imagery to represent the chaos that the ER must deal with every day of the year, the absurdity that can come through the sliding glass doors from the parking lot at any moment—absurdities that demand immediate, professional, and exact medical response. One day the radio informed us that seven migrant workers were being brought to the ER. They had taken shelter under a truck during a storm, and the truck was struck by lightning. The ER had to take this, or any other chaotic event, in stride.

Freudian Attack

Fluffy and Snowball also represent the anger and stress that caregivers feel from the demands of their work. The results of their work can make a patient well or sicker, can cure or kill—and few professionals are so closely watched. Mistakes can yield an "incident report," which can lead to the disciplining or dismissal of the healthcare worker. Doctors or nurses can be sued for malpractice; they can lose their licenses and therefore ways to use the skills they took years to master. Nurses, in particular, must deal with deranged, disgusting, or unruly patients. The doctors can come and go, but it falls to nurses to be responsible minute by minute, hour by hour, for every patient in the ER. And all ER workers, whether medical or clerical, see suffering in patients and feel, in the traditional phrase, "There but for the grace of God go I." The rabid Fluffy is an analogue for sick patients, every accident, every illness that might occur to any of us at any time; the Fluffy game is an exercise in playful control.

In fact, there is no real control over evil, only a sense of play that affirms the freedom of the Fluffy players, even while they check and recheck meds, patients' name bracelets, lab results, and update the patient's chart, the medical and legal document that is central to delivery of care. One of the ways the chart was put together was lavish use of the copy machine. (This was still true in the 1990s, the time of my story; charts in hospitals now are more and more paperless, created at computer terminals.) The photocopying of the Fluffy material was a form of rebellion, an unauthorized use of hospital resources, we might say, or, more positively, raising the status of the machine from servile utility to something more creative and imaginative. In this way, office materials and structures are, depending on your point of view, rebelliously subverted or creatively and comically redeemed.

DEATH MORE THAN SEX

This is not the erotic Green World of some hospital humor. Of all the exhibits, few have sexual themes (the condom advertisement; the house pets' hot date), and only Cinderella suggests an idealized female figure; the missing child parody obliquely ties into the comic theme of having a future generation. Rather, the world of Fluffy and Snowball is dominated by violent imagery that is manipulated playfully. Such playfulness is an expression of freedom for ER workers to go beyond their normal limits of behavior, thoughts, and emotions. The subject matter of vicious dogs may be read as a psychodrama to represent the suffering of patients who arrive at the ER with all sorts of absurd and dangerous injuries. In the ER, pain, loss of function, disfigurement, and death are common and always a possibility, any hour of the day or night. The rebellion of using office materials and the playfulness of manipulating the images of Fluffy and Snowball suggest a domestication of evil and a statement about creative freedom in an exacting and difficult milieu that requires strict discipline.

RITUALS AND COMMUNITIES

The emotional content is pretty clear. Instead of disgust, depression, or anger at the chaos of the ER (and the world in general), the Fluffy game makes fun of these, provides for laughter, and gives a feeling of freedom.

In terms of communities, there were three: (1) the comic community of the Fluffy players, (2) the non-comic hospital administration—who could ignore the game, at least for a while, either because they didn't know about it or because they saw no risks involved, and (3) the indeterminate but surely non-comic community of patients and their families. The last group, of course, would be the risky group, since they wouldn't know the language, the moods, or the social benefits. If I'm taking a family member to an ER, the last thing I want to see are cartoons of rabid dogs.

Comic communities work best when they are well defined and when the members agree on some basic norms for humor. When I was in college, Black students could make jokes about themselves that white students dared not make, Jewish students could joke about Jews in ways WASPS wouldn't. Some of the ER personnel had nothing to do with the Fluffy game, and I imagine it's possible that some of them didn't like it. Among the Fluffy players, however, there was a camaraderie, a shared language and values. Furthermore, this community was highly democratic. Ordinarily, there is a hierarchy of hospital personnel in authority (and power and earnings) from top administration to doctors, to middle managers, to nurses, to clerks, to techs, to housekeeping personnel, with volunteers at the bottom. With the Fluffy game, however, anyone could play, and all, at least in theory, would be equally accepted. When actual people—whether doctors or nurses—were named in the doctored photos, they were equally invited to join in the Fluffy game.

If we compare the Party Time! humor to the Fluffy game, there are some large differences, especially in mood and materials used. In Party Time! the ritual occurred person-to-person with the opening of the restraint drawer. In Fluffy, the postings were anonymous, to be viewed by others later, even on other shifts. In Party Time! the joking dealt specifically with the emotionally difficult subject of restraints, while in Fluffy the jokers had a wide range of subjects, materials, changes to texts, making masks, and so on. In Party Time! there was a Freudian counter-attack to the sad duty of using restraints, while in Fluffy there was an open field of play for office humor, all starting with a single image from a book about rabies, a dangerous disease that was left far, far behind.

Chapter Twelve

"Smile When You Say That, Mister"

Conclusions About Clowns and Jokers

ONE DAY MY boss suggested I take my massage chair up to the Pediatric Oncology Unit, where the staff was under some stress. Between my morning rounds, I got permission from an attending physician, Stuart Gold, and showed up after lunch pulling my chair on its wheels. This unit is on the second floor of the brand new North Carolina Cancer Hospital, a $220 million building with hotel-like design. The Peds unit has bright colors, big windows, and, at child height, large posters of animals on the doors of the exam rooms. Dr. Gold showed me to the Orangutan room, where I could set up.

When I came back to the nurses' area, he introduced me to a nurse, suggesting I offer chair massage to her, although, he warned, "You'll definitely need to mask and triple-glove."

What? I thought, looking at his face to get a reading of his intent. I could see only a poker face. I'd heard of double-gloving against dangerous pathogens, but never triple-gloving—a strong clue.

Then his right eye winked, an even stronger clue that he was joking.

"Do you carry Hanta virus?" I asked her.

"Oh yes," she said, "among several others."

I offered massage, she accepted, and back we went to the Orangutan room.

Was this a test to see if I could fit into the Peds brand of humor? An invitation? A rite of passage? Whatever the ritual, it enabled me to understand that there was a comic community within the professional community that treated sick children.

HUMOROUS HUMANS;
MAXIMAL BENEFITS AND HARMS OF HUMOR

Although most professionals assume rational inquiry is (and should be) paramount, humans use humor a lot, even delighting in its irrationality. Such humor ranges from silly puns to earthy humor; indeed, the name "human" has the same root as the word "humus."

Humor is a basic and undeniable feature of human behavior, but it can have differing uses: it can provide a powerful resource for creating and maintaining communities, or a distraction, or a hurtful weapon. Recalling terms from the Cloud of Aspirations and the Solid Footings in Chapter Four, we can consider that one maximal benefit of humor is Freedom, which suggests power, choice, and opportunity—values well in tune with successful comedy and humor. But the negative side of freedom can be lack of order, anomie, even panic at being unmoored and adrift. A maximal harm of humor is Anarchy or lack of order that leads to Chaos. The conventions of comedy avoid such harm by providing social rituals, comic communities, traditional values, and familiar literary elements, all Solid Footings in their own right.

The other maximal benefit is, in its optimal form, the notion of Gift, but there is also an opposite, which is Assault (as in "assault and battery," the legal phrase for verbal threat and physical touch).

FIGURE 12.1: MAXIMAL BENEFITS AND HARMS OF HUMOR

HUMOR AS	BENEFIT OR HARM
Freedom	Green World
Anarchy	Chaos
Gift	Green World
Assault	Chaos

Our final chapter has three parts: (1) a summary of the main points, (2) testing the gifts and dangers of humor, and (3) practical applications for the world of medicine and beyond.

IN SUMMARY

In this study my first aim was to describe the many ways in which comedy and humor occur, both in emergent humor (as in vignettes from hospitals and clinics) and also in the oral tradition of jokes. We've seen differences in tone from the gentle humor of the hospital clown Vonnie to the raucous, even bawdy humor of the ER. While hospitals and clinics are clearly places with serious work to do, there is also a lot of humor within them and also much humor outside about them; both kinds of humor reflect our intense interest, concern, and fears about disease and death, as well as the affirmations (sometimes indirect) we make about life itself.

My second aim was to analyze the elements of humor, using literary terms and concepts (largely Chapters Five through Nine). We can now expand Figure 4.5, the Overview of Comic Features from Chapter Four.

FIGURE 12.2: OVERVIEW OF COMIC FEATURES EXPANDED

Primary Character	Audience	Tone	Style	Underlying Metaphor	Healing Purpose
Vonnie (Clown)	Hospital patients (Asymetrical)	Gentle	Improv Comedy	Circus (Festive escape)	Comfort
Party Time! (Joker, very strong)	ER coworkers (Symmetrical)	Harsh	Code	Erotic bondage (Sexual escape)	Ironic solidarity Coping with stress
Jokes (via email) (Joker, weak)	Social peers at leisure (Symmetrical but distant)	Varies	Written	Verbal play (Literary escape)	Pleasure Entertainment
Jokes (spoken) (Joker, strong or weak)	Social peers at leisure (Symmetrical and present)	Varies	Oral	Verbal play (Literary performance Social escape)	Pleasure Entertainment Social ritual
"Explanations of Hospital Policy" (Joker/writer, strong)	Anyone on the Net	Freudian attack	Parody	Unfair rules of hospital deserve scorn, ridicule	Shared vengeance Moral order Hilarity
Pearly Gate Jokes (Joker/writer)	Anyone on the Net	Mixed	Allegory	Life and afterlife have a moral basis	Laughter about death
Brunhilde in ICU (Anonymous hospital worker)	Anyone in the ICU, including visitors	Playful	Visual	Hospital equipment personified	Playfulness, even in an ICU

This figure is schematic, suggestive of major features while ignoring variations and subtleties. The range of humor in Chapters Eight, Nine, and Ten is too wide for a reductive formulation, so I've picked three examples. The elaborate parody "Explanations of Hospital Policy" will serve as a Freudian attack; such attacks illustrate the human need to vent anger (catharsis) as well as to express strongly held values. The Pearly Gates jokes suggest our instincts for survival, our culture's difficulties with death, the symbol of sex to represent vitality, and questions about moral lives and the ultimate worth of our souls. Brunhilde in the ICU will serve as an example of office humor.

As in the earlier Figure 4.6, Overview Flat on the Table, two off-the-chart features lie above and below Figure 12.2: the Cloud of Aspirations (Freedom, Agency, and Joy) and the Solid Footings (Social Solidarity, Sex, Comfort, Entertainment, and Pleasure). Each area has positive and negative aspects. (We looked at Freedom vs. Anarchy a few paragraphs back.) The phrase "Solid Footings" sounds positive, as for a building, but it could also suggest boring homogeneity. Pleasure can be escapist and/or decadent, and Earthy humor may or may not be acceptable; too much dirt or animalism may suggest a pigsty or worse, and a need for uplifting Levity. Taken together, Levity and Gravity are two contradictory aspects of humor that help create comic activity. Comedy, we might say, outflanks normalcy by going above and below it, giving a wider context for how we live our lives.

The third aim was to consider the social utility of comic behavior: how much does comedy help? It depends. In some situations jokes and laughter are not appropriate. There are times when the mood or culture or frame of reference of the joker and others are not similar, and the joke falls flat or even insults people. To maintain wholeness and continuity and not offend, comedy needs consistency of mood and agreement of the participating community. Comedy can be an adjunct to medicine by (1) helping us name the things that trouble us, (2) exploring and changing their meanings and our emotional responses, (3) suggesting control of them or freedom from them, (4) exercising our imaginations, (5) enhancing our sense of agency and freedom, and (6) creating supportive comic communities. Especially in medical settings, the rituals and conventions of comedy help to humanize encounters between patients and caregivers by reminding patients of social bonds that suggest equality and solidarity with well persons. Through comedy we belong to the world of the well, even if we are sick.

Like the contradictory Levity and Gravity, the "crazy logic" of jokes arises from the rational and irrational elements that make up the comedic experience. We have seen this experience symbolized by the Green World, a hypothetical world that provides a counterpoint to the music (or noise) of mundane life, the Work-A-Day World dominated by duty, performance norms, utility, linear causality, profit/loss calculations, net worth, pecking order, and the like. This is the heritage of Euclid, Aristotle, Newton, John Stuart Mill, and all positivists and rationalists in general. All of these influences are important, assuredly, and pillars of the modern world, but we do not live by syllogisms alone. Humor deals with, expresses, cultivates, and frees up our emotions, our intuitions, and our instincts.

Testing For Dangers Of Comedy

We may imagine humor as a force like an energy wave that may aid or destroy, depending on the application, the intent, and the setting. How can we tell whether humor is positive or negative? Given all the variables involved in people and settings, it would be futile to make up universal rules, but I'll suggest four tests that individuals and groups might use to assess appropriateness.

1. To What Extent Is There a Comic Community?

The first test harks back to a list under "Dilemmas in Appropriateness" in Chapter Four. Do all the participants have similar senses of humor, or might some be offended? Even if there is sufficient agreement on humor, is the timing right, or is the mood too somber, or the workload too pressing? Is someone present being scapegoated? Is someone absent being scapegoated unfairly or even slanderously? Are newcomers or the least powerful protected?

2. Does the Humor Show Kind Intention?

"Smile when you say that, Mister" is a cliché from Westerns; its origin is Owen Wister's novel *The Virginian* (1902), which was made into several movies.[1] In those settings, the phrase is ironic, even hostile, but we ordinarily consider a smile positively as an indicator of kind intent. Like the doctor's wink, a smile symbolizes person-to-person kindness that is a positive emotional context for whatever words are spoken. In broad terms, humor can show three kinds of intention: (A) kind intention, such as the wish to entertain, cheer up, or give pleasure, (B) satiric intention to criticize persons or institutions and correct them according to positive values, and (C) attacking humor that intends to degrade, punish, or reject a person, an institution, or an ideal. Our emphasis in this book is on types A and B. Type A is especially well suited to hospital, clinics, and sickrooms in general where there are marked differences between the sick and the well. Types A and B can be helpful in the world of the well where people make jokes. Type C can entertain and/or engender conflict, perhaps with tragic results, perhaps with positive changes, or both.

Kind intention helps us understand the next two tests of Freedom and Gift.

3. Does the Humor Enhance the Freedom of Others?

The humor of the hospital clown Vonnie helped patients feel free for several reasons: she helped them laugh at or forget their troubles, she provided reminders of the experience of the circus, she responded positively to anything patients said so that they could express their feelings freely, and she offered cheerful banter with jokes. While Vonnie didn't heal patients' illness or free them from their rooms, she helped them experience freedom from such emotions as sadness, loneliness, and boredom. She helped them feel free in their imaginations through the specific metaphor of the circus and, more generally, through the attributes of a Green World where good things routinely happen. Taking patients' minds away from their troubles is an aspect of healing.

If we assume that the humor of Party Time! worked for the nurses involved, some of its power came from freeing nurses from the dread and guilt of tying up patients and also from affirming their responsibility in performing nurses' duties.

Harmful humor is annoying and distracting from more important concerns. It can be a source of anarchy because it lacks the mood of kind intention and agreement of a community. Ideally, a person considering making a joke in any setting might first ask, "Is it my intention that this joke helps the listeners feel happy and free?"

4. Is the Humor a Gift?

Much of human behavior is governed by exchanges of goods and services on a quid-pro-quo basis. Accordingly, gifts can be suspect because we wonder if there's a hidden agenda: what does the given expect in return? The Trojan Horse is a famous example of a gift with hidden costs.

If a joke is offered, it should have the intention of giving pleasure to others and deepening the social connections. It should be free of hidden costs, such as the joker's wish to be idolized because of brilliance in performing.

These four tests can help individuals or groups assess whether humor is appropriate.

Gifts In The Worlds Of Medical Treatment

We go to the doctor and, if we are lucky, the receptionist smiles and says, "How are you?" While taking our weight and vital signs, the nurse smiles, uses our name, and pats us on the arm. The doctor says, "Sorry you had to wait, but thanks for coming. It sure was cold this morning, wasn't it?" None of these actions are, "medically necessary," in the legal phrase. They do not contribute to analyzing the patient's "chief complaint," finding the diagnosis, or making a treatment plan. Rather, they are gifts, free and clear, from one person to another, with no cost, no codes for diagnosis or implications for billing and insurance. Nonetheless, they are powerful and valuable, because they contribute to a patient's wellbeing by recognizing him or her as a fellow human being. Such ritual greetings may seem ephemeral, but they establish a caring context for medical care and assurances to patients that, however ill or injured they may be, they are still human beings worthy of respect. A paradox emerges: such activities are not the main business, but they are very important, even priceless.

Why are gifts so powerful? As opposed to wages or debts, gifts are not earned or required. They come for free, regardless of whether we deserve them. Gifts suggest that the giver is generous and has the intentions of kindness toward us and the aim to help us or give us pleasure. Emergent humor such as Brunhilde in the ICU or jokes emailed from a friend come out of the blue, unexpected and unearned. Dictionaries tell us that the Latin root *gratus* or "pleasing" has evolved in English to several related words, including "gratis" (for free), "gratuity" (a tip to a waiter), even "grace," as in John Bunyan's *Grace Abounding to the Chief of Sinners* or John Newton's famous "Amazing Grace." Although these words all have positive connotations, another related word, "gratuitous," does not. Humor is gratuitous when it is unwelcome and unjustifiable.

In times past, the Good Humor Man drove around neighborhoods selling ice cream. This brilliant piece of marketing suggested that he (or she) brought not only ice cream but also good humor to everyone, energizing entire neighborhoods. This is the realm of gentle jokers, people who don't tell jokes per se but who are polite, kind, and willing to relate to other people, even strangers, and make them feel welcome. Earlier we called them "smilers."

At the heart of comedy and humor is the kind intention that makes possible the maximal benefits of happiness and freedom. Such intention is expressed by words, gestures, or touches that (1) give a sense of freedom from the limitations of the world (including pain, loneliness, and fear) and that (2) offer the ritual of giving a gift that suggests that the recipients are worthy of love and being embraced within a society of social equals.

SOURCES OF LACK OF HUMOR

We might think that the gracious acts of the receptionist, nurse, and doctor just described would be automatic, part of common courtesy, and universally occurring. Why aren't they?

Common courtesy has had a difficult time in the last few decades. Modern, urban life in America is increasingly stressed, stressing, and distressing. Cities, highways, malls, and airports are all more crowded. Commuting is tedious. Although many people are ambitious, many are not making economic gains. Terrorism, warfare, economic collapse, pollution, Global Warming, and nasty politics dominate the headlines and provide an unpleasant context for daily life. There is unemployment and underemployment. According to polls, job dissatisfaction is common. Aging Baby Boomers confront their mortality. There are pervasive signs of withdrawal (cocooning) and narcissism: people closed off in their cars, homes, "gated communities" (literally a paradoxical phrase, emphasizing the exclusion of others), in the worlds of their cell phones and other electronic devices, in their "full calendars" and "electronic social networks"—all to the suppression of direct, leisurely engagement with other people. I fear this is a distinctly American problem, since Americans commonly believe in their exceptionalism, their city on the hill, their land of opportunity from sea to shining sea: go west, young man and be the new Horatio Alger, because every boy/girl can be president. One study ranks the US as "the world's 23rd happiest nation, behind countries such as Costa Rica, Malta, and Malaysia."[2] Even ranking is a national obsession and many people/teams/institutions desperately desire to be Number One! because we consider Number Two (or lower!) to be a grotesque failure. Furthermore, there are larger and larger income disparities in the US, and, for many people, free-floating anger and hopelessness. Traditional societies, with much less money, are often happier. Hasan and Hasan have studied laughter in an Indian city and a Canadian city, concluding that individualist cultures—such as ours, with more personal emotions—have less life satisfaction than do collectivist cultures—such as in India, with more reliance on group interests—and, therefore, different uses of humor.[3]

Contemporary Americans, although meaning to be friendly (and often considering themselves very friendly), often do not have time or the focus or the energy to act in friendly ways.

What are some of the causes for lack of humor in medical offices? The tasks themselves may not require being friendly with patients; after all, medicine is an applied science and the job is to assess, diagnose, and treat as rationally as possible. The commonly used SOAP notes specify categories for an orderly assessment: Subjective comments of the patient, Objective notes of the observer, Assessment or diagnoses, and Plan, or what to do; I'd suggest a new acronym, GSOAP, with a human-to-human Greeting heading the list. There are two recent books with the same title, *How Doctors Think*, but where are the books entitled *How Doctors Laugh with Patients* or *How Doctors Are Social with Patients?*[4]

Medical staff may be overworked because of too many patients, long hours (some nurses work 12-hour shifts), even double shifts. Tasks may be so routine as to be boring over months, years, even decades. Workers may see no hope of career development; they may feel job fatigue or burnout. Staff may be so used to close focus on tasks as to forget about the wider context of human relationships with patients, even the larger purpose of healthcare, to support the wellbeing of fellow humans and society in general. If you work 40 hours a week in medical care, seeing the same sorts of health problems over and over, it may be hard to understand how a particular patient feels about a distressing illness or injury that is mysterious and frightening.

Here is a real-life story (with some changes and also thanks to the woman who shared it):

Lack Of Laughter In A Veterinarian's Office
My cat was progressively sicker all day. I kept hoping he'd snap out of it, but as the evening wore on, he seemed no better. About midnight, I felt he was decidedly worse, so I called the vet's office, and an on-call vet agreed to meet me there.

When I took the cat in, I was quite concerned, or maybe frantic would be a better term. The vet looked him over and said, "He's pretty sick; you'll have to leave him here."

"You're not going to torture him?" I joked.

He turned red and stiffly replied, "Madam, remarks such as those do not exactly endear you to this office."

I was stunned. I was already distraught about the cat, but then I had to drive home feeling rejected as well by the very person I trusted to help me.

Of course she was stunned. She made a joke with the extreme image of torture that indirectly expressed her inner fear about her cat. Certainly the vet should have known that owners are routinely fearful about their very sick pets and should have understood the emotional truth behind her strange question, an invitation for him to join her in a comic community, to help change the emotions of the moment, and to include her as a social equal through the ritual of a shared joke. Instead he cut her off, clearly and tragically making her a humiliated outsider.

Who knows why he acted in such an inappropriate way? The only clue I see from this written version is the word "office," suggesting that he saw himself in an official, bureaucratic role and not as a person offering services to animals and people. Furthermore, he apparently did not recognize that it's common for patients to initiate humor in medical settings; one study found that when there was humor between Hospice patients and nurses, seventy percent of the time it was patients who initiated it.[5]

What might he have said instead? One route would be to join in the exact idiom of her humor, although this would probably be too harsh: "Oh yes, we have a special room for that." Better would be, "There will certainly be no torture of this fine kitty; it has been through enough already." Or he could speak to the emotions that her joke indirectly expressed: "I know you're very concerned about this cat, and we'll do our very best to take care of it."

How's the Weather Now?

One day in a clinic, I overheard a doctor ask a patient, "How's the weather now?" The patient was a bit surprised, suddenly an authority on something the doctor didn't know about because the doctor had been at work all day inside. The patient explained about the temperature, amount of sunshine, and the like, glad to be of service. For that moment, the doctor and patient were social equals, both in the world of the well before entering into the healthcare transaction that would make their roles unequal.

To speculate further, we could say "weather" also meant an ambient mood of doctor and patient, thus emphasizing their common humanity before turning to other, common questions such as "What brings you here today?" "How are you feeling?" "Did those pills give you any relief?" At the level of a comforting ritual, the patient might have felt, "The weather is good today because you greeted me as a fellow human." We're stretching the notion of comedy here beyond jokes and laughter; this is the smiling realm of caring intention, and it is quite powerful. In the world of the sick, comedy can create a context for the delivery of medicine that is nourishing to patient and caregiver alike. In the world of the well, we tell jokes to shape the "weather" surrounding medical topics that bother us, a widely practiced (if somewhat strange) form of preventive medicine.

Healing Can Contribute to Curing

Good uses of humor can have positive impacts on patients, even a gesture as simple as the smile and touch of the Jamaican man we saw in Chapter Four. These were signs of loving intention that reached something deep in the woman near death, thereby giving her a sense of wholeness and health. The word "heal" relates to other words such as, "holy," "whole," and "hale," all concepts of blessedness, integrity, and vitality. The Jamaican man was, in some miraculous way, a messenger from the Green World, bringing his improbable and unexpected gift of healing. Whether health professionals or lay folk, we can bring the humor of the Green World to the sick, whether they are getting well, dying, or in a limbo that seems to go on forever.

When we are sick, we have time to reflect on our previous healthy life, a life that may seem much greener when we're on the other side of the fence. We count our blessings and hope to recover them. We may also feel neglected and tragically separated (in Frye's sense) from our desired society. Any hints of connection to the Green World are most welcome, and the sick person often values them highly, well beyond any estimation of the giver. Maybe it's food, some flowers, a card, a book, a phone call. Any of these may seem a hundred times more powerful to the recipient than to the giver. Such tokens are signs of the Green World of the well, symbols that the sick person still belongs to that world, embraced by a comic community.

APPLICATIONS FOR COMEDY AND MEDICINE

In this section we turn to my fourth aim, practical ways we can improve the delivery of medical care, deal with illness in others, and care for our own health.

AMONG CAREGIVERS

Medical people often use humor, even though outsiders may perceive them as "all business." In-house, in-group humor can range from the playfulness of Brunhilde in the ICU to the bawdy humor of Party Time! This backstage or offstage humor can entertain, relieve tension, create social bonds, and add playfulness to a stressful milieu. Humor, however, that leads to or reinforces callousness toward patients (or other staff) is not helpful. If a member of a group relentlessly uses humor that is unseemly, a colleague or supervisor should point out that this behavior can have a negative influence in the workplace. Possibly the joker is unaware of the impact and inappropriateness of his or her humor.

If there are guests at a conference or rounds, there is further complexity, because shared norms cannot be taken for granted. Perhaps the humor should be dampened or omitted for that day, or the leader might say that the group sometimes uses humor and explain why it is helpful. This could be important to students in medical training. If the guests are non-medical, further discretion and sensitivity would be advisable.

Frank discussion in medical schools and residency programs about positive and negative uses of humor may also be helpful. Does our humor support our work, relieve our stress, deepen bonds with each other, and help us care for our patients? Do we offer humor to other personnel and to our patients in supportive ways?

BETWEEN CAREGIVERS AND PATIENTS

In modern times, we often forget that a hospital is supposed to be a hospitable place; both words have French and Latin roots meaning "receiving guests, as a host."

Modern hospital designs look more and more like hotels and spas, with atriums, pretty colors, art, window views—all with an aim of helping patients to feel "at home" and lessening their anxiety. When I went through orientation (with about 200 nurses) for my massage job at University of North Carolina Hospitals, one of the speakers specifically said that it was part of our job to treat patients as if they were guests in our own homes. The floor nurses I see are routinely polite and considerate to patients. Chaplains and social workers are specifically charged with helping patients with issues beyond the strictly medical dilemmas, and kindness is central to their work. Recreational therapists help patients with activities that will cheer them up, and we've seen the work of hospital clown Vonnie.

MEDICALLY NECESSARY HUMOR: CHECKLISTS, TRAINING, EXPECTATIONS

Recent news reports about healthcare reform have mentioned checklists as a measure that cuts costs by lessening medical errors; President Obama spoke about checklists on TV. Atul Gawande's book *The Checklist Manifesto: How to Get Things Right* tells how medicine has learned from aviation (US Army Air Corps pilots in the 1930s, as well as the Boeing Company) that checklists can decrease errors and improve efficiency.[6] I saw a "Competency Checklist" in an oncology setting entitled "Removal of Non-Tunneled Central Venous Catheter." It includes twenty-two items from No. 1. ("Verifies in patient's chart for provider order, presence of bleeding disorders or clinical precautions") all the way through to No. 22, specifying documentation. These are technical steps, surely all necessary, but I think No. 1 should be some version of "Greets patient in a friendly fashion, establishes rapport, and explains procedure briefly."

As with the justification for brand name drugs instead of generics—that they are medically necessary—treating fellow humans as fellow humans should routinely be medically necessary. This should be an absolute performance goal, reinforced by checklists, in-service training, evaluations, or whatever bureaucratic encouragements are needed. Patients should expect no less. Caregivers would have happier days. More people would get well and stay well.

IN THE WORLD OF THE WELL

There's a bumper sticker with a picture of a dog and the exhortation, "BARK LESS, WAG MORE."

I would recommend that people enjoy humor more, seeking it out, using it, and delighting in it. We often work too hard and act too seriously and competitively. Humor is a stress-reducer. Humor brings joy. Humor deepens friendships and can enrich even casual social interactions.

MASSAGE, BLOODY MARYS, AND CERTIFICATES IN THE INFUSION ROOM

A half a dozen years after my own chemotherapy, I enter an infusion room once again. This time I'm not a patient about to sit in a chair for four, five, or six hours, receiving medicine from a pump through a needle inserted into my hand. Instead, I'm a licensed massage therapist, with added training in massage for hospital patients in general and cancer patients in particular. I approach a patient receiving treatment and say, "Hi there. My name is Howard, and I'm a massage therapist. I can massage your hands or your feet while you're receiving treatment." Some patients (often men) say, "I'm fine" and decline. Others say, "Yes," especially if I've massaged them before or if they've seen me massaging another patient nearby. I sit on a wheeled stool in front of their Barcalounger and massage their hands with lotion or, after taking off shoes and socks, their feet.

On my chest I wear a plastic badge—white letters on a green background—that reads CANCER SURVIVOR. About eighty percent of my patients ask me about it. Much as I needed a symbol of life beyond cancer—which I found in the woman who had lost her hair three times—patients want to know about my status: what kind did I have, what treatment, how long ago, and how do I feel now? One man pointed to my badge and said, "Gosh, I sure hope to be one of those someday!" I replied, to his surprise and delight, "You're a survivor right now, in fact from the minute you were diagnosed." He straightened up in his chair, murmuring, "I'm a survivor, I'm a survivor."

Often patients receiving chemo don't know each other and stay quiet. As I massage and talk with one of them, however, wider conversations often start up including nearby patients. Sometimes it's humor that makes the links. When a nurse comes with a medication or to adjust an IV pump, I say, "Hey, we'd like a couple of Bloody Marys here." The nurses know my style and reply, "Coming right up," "Singles or doubles?" or "Great, and I'll have one too." Sometimes patients chime in, "Me too, and I'd like extra spices," while another calls out, "Two celeries for me!" and we all laugh.

We have described people using humor as jokers, who range from the most extreme wisecrackers to conventional clowns and gentle smilers. Comedy provides familiar structures and rituals, both in the forms of humor and in themes. When jokers match up with audiences sharing similar values and expectations, there is a social

solidarity that is satisfying and healing. If topics include difficult subject matter—
such as illness, the limits of our bodies, even death—there is a psychological comfort
in knowing that fellow humans are troubled by the same topics.

It is my hope that this study contributes to the ongoing humanization of healthcare in hospitals and clinics and, in the worlds of the well, to our understanding of
how comedy (and humor) can serve as an imaginative and energizing form of preventive medicine.

On a patient's last day of chemotherapy, oncology nurses arrive clapping rhyth-
mically and singing, "For s/he's a jolly good fellow." They wave a musical wand over
the patient's head and give her or him a handsomely printed Certificate of Achievement with a lovely engraved blue border and a large purple heart; it reads:

CERTIFICATE OF ACHIEVEMENT
UNC HEMATOLOGY/ONCOLOGY STAFF
PRESENTS THIS
PURPLE HEART AWARD
TO
[NAME]
FOR COURAGEOUSLY COMPLETING
CHEMOTHERAPY!

The patient is glad for several reasons, and other patients watch with pleasure,
thinking of the time when their chemotherapy will also be over. For many patients,
this is the end of treatment; they are in remission or even entirely cured. For others,
the chemo was to shrink the tumor so that surgery would go more easily. Some patients have been treated for a recurrence, which may happen yet again. Still others are
going home to die, perhaps under Hospice care or to a Hospice facility.

Whatever comes next, patients have received from the nurses a comic blessing, a
ritual that exemplifies kind intention and offers both Freedom and Gift.

Endnotes

Introduction

1 Jim Holt, *Stop Me if You've Heard This: A History and Philosophy of Jokes* (New York: W. W. Norton, 2008).

2 Ivan Illich, *Medical Nemesis: The Expropriation of Health* (New York: Random House, 1976).

3 Albert Howard Carter, III, *First Cut: A Season in the Human Anatomy Lab* (New York: Picador, 1997), *Rising from the Flames: The Experience of the Severely Burned*, with Jane Arbuckle Petro (Philadelphia: Univ. of Pennsylvania Press, 1998), and *Our Human Hearts: A Medical and Cultural Journey* (Kent, Ohio: Kent State Univ. Press, 2006).

4 Richard Hooker, *Mash* (New York: Morrow, 1968).

5 Samuel Shem, *House of God: A Novel* (New York: R. Marek Pubs., 1978).

6 Norman Cousins, *Anatomy of an Illness as Perceived by the Patient: Reflections on Healing and Regeneration* (New York: W.W. Norton, 1979).

7 Patch Adams, with Maureen Mylander, *Gesundheit!* (Rochester, Vt.: Healing Arts Press, 1998) and *House Calls: How We Can Heal the World One Visit at a Time* (Bandon, Ore.: Robert D. Reed Publishers, 1998).

8 Sokichi Sakuragi, Yoshiki Sugiyama, Kiyomi Takeuchi, "Effects of Laughing and Weeping on Mood and Heart Rate Variability," *Journal of Physiological Anthropology* 21.3 (2002): 159-165.

9 M. Gervais and D.S. Wilson, "The Evolution and Functions of Laughter and Humor: A Synthetic Approach," *Quarterly Review of Biology* 80.4 (2005): 395-430.

10 C. Hassad, "How Humour Keeps You Well," *Australian Family Physician* 30.1 (2001): 25-28; Hélène Patenaude, Louis Hamelin Brabant, "L'Humour dans la Relation Infirmière-Patient: Une Revue de la Littérature" *Recherche en Soins Infirmiers* 85 (2006): 36-45. See also M.P. Zeller et al., "The Effect of Mirthful Laughter on Stress and Natural Killer Cell Activity," *Alternative Therapies in Health and Medicine* 9.2 (2003): 38-45 and Adam Clark et al., "Inverse Association between Sense of Humor and Coronary Heart Disease," *International Journal of Cardiology* 80 (2001): 87-88.

11 Mary Payne Bennett and Cecile Lengacher, "Humor and Laughter May Influence Health: II," Complementary Therapies and Humor in a Clinical Population," 3.2

(2006): 187-190. [PubMed]. See also C. Hassad, "How Humour Keeps You Well," *Australian Family Physician* 30.1 (2001): 25-28.

12 Anne Hudson Jones, "Narrative in Medical Ethics," *British Medical Journal* 318 (January 23, 1999): 253-256.

13 *Literature and Medicine* 13.1 (1994): 79-92.

14 Anne Hunsaker Hawkins, *Reconstructing Illness: Studies in Pathography* (West Lafayette: Purdue Univ. Press, 1992), Kathryn Montgomery Hunter, *Doctors' Stories: The Narrative Structure of Medical Knowledge* (Princeton: Princeton Univ. Press, 1991), Kathryn Montgomery, *How Doctors Think: Clinical Judgment and the Practice of Medicine* (New York: Oxford Univ. Press, 2006), Rita Charon, *Narrative Medicine: Honoring the Stories of Illness* (New York: Oxford Univ. Press, 2006), and Paul C. Horton, *Solace: The Missing Dimension in Psychiatry* (Chicago: Univ. of Chicago Press, 1981).

15 Vera Kalizkus and Peter F. Matthiessen, "Narrative-Based Medicine: Potential, Pitfalls, and Practice," *Permanente Journal* 13.1 (2009): 80-86.

16 Jeffrey P. Bishop, "Rejecting Medical Humanism: Medical Humanities and the Metaphysics of Medicine," *Journal of Medical Humanities* 10 (2008): 15-25.

17 Jeff Rowin, *500 Great Doctor Jokes* (New York: Signet, 1993) is simply a listing of many jokes. In another, more academic book, Che Prasad approaches jokes about doctors using concepts from folklore and psychology in *Physician Humor Thyself: An Analysis of Doctor Jokes* (Winston-Salem: Harbinger Medical Press, 1998); Prasad limits his discussion to jokes about specific medical specialties, such as primary care, surgery, dermatology, etc.

Chapter One

1 Northrop Frye, *Anatomy of Criticism* (Princeton, Princeton Univ. Press, 1957).

2 Joseph Campbell, *The Hero with A Thousand Faces*. 1949; rpt. rev. ed. (Princeton Univ. Press, 1968).

3 Susan Sontag, *Illness as Metaphor* and *AIDS and Its Metaphors* (New York: Picador, 1989).

4 Eric J. Cassell, *The Healer's Art* (Cambridge: MIT Press, 1985).

5 Barbara G. Kruse and Mark Prazak "Humor and Older Adults: What Makes them Laugh," *Journal of Holistic Nursing* 24 (2006): 188-193, 192.

6 Hunald Hasan and Tasneem Fatema Hasan, "Laugh Yourself into a Healthier Person: A Cross Cultural Analysis of the Effects of Varying Levels of Laughter on Health,"

International Journal of Medical Sciences 6(4) (2009): 200-211.

7 Cesar Lombardy Barber, *Shakespeare's Festive Comedy: A Study of Dramatic Form and Its Relation to Social Custom* (Princeton: Princeton Univ. Press, 1959).

8 Edward O. Wilson, *Biophilia* (Cambridge, Mass.: Harvard Univ. Press, 1984).

9 Gaston Bachelard, *The Poetics of Space.* Trans. Maria Jolas. (Boston: Beacon, 1969).

10 Kathryn Montgomery Hunter, *Doctors' Stories: The Narrative Structure of Medical Knowledge* (Princeton, NJ: Princeton Univ. Press, 1991) and Rita Charon's *Narrative Medicine: Honoring the Stories of Illness* (Oxford, New York: Oxford Univ. Press, 2006).

11 Kathryn Montgomery, *How Doctors Think: Clinical Judgment and the Practice of Medicine* (Oxford, New York: Oxford Univ. Press, 2006).

Chapter Two

1 Alexander Solzhenitsyn, *Cancer Ward.* Translated by Nicholas Bethell and David Burg. (New York: Modern Library, 1983).

2 Albert Howard Carter, III, "Literary Analogues to Living Wills," in *Advance Directives in Medicine,* eds. Chris Hackler, Ray Mosley, and Dorothy E. Vawter. (New York: Praeger, 1987): 181-87.

3 Elisabeth Kübler-Ross, *On Death and Dying* (New York: Macmillan, 1969).

4 Jean-Dominique Bauby, *The Diving Bell and the Butterfly.* Trans. Jeremy Leggatt. (New York: Knopf, 1997).

5 Barbara Wald et al., "Clowns in der Psychiatrie? Ein Pilotprojekt," *Nervenarzt* 78.5 (June 2007): 571-74, and L. Vagnoli, S. Caprilli, A. Robiglio, and A. Messeri, "Clown Doctors as a Treatment for Preoperative Anxiety in Children: A Randomized, Prospective Study," *Pediatrics* 116.4 (2005): 563-7.

6 Selena Clare McMahan, "Infinite Possibility: Clowning with Elderly People," *Care Management Journals* 9.1 (2008): 19-24, p. 22.

7 McMahan, p. 23.

8 McMahan, p. 23.

Chapter Three

1 W. Maxwell, "The Use of Gallows Humor and Dark Humor During Crisis Situations," *International Journal of Emergency Mental Health* 5.2 (2003): 93-98.

2 Lee and Bob Woodruff, *In an Instant: A Family's Journey of Love and Healing* (New York: Random House, 2007).

3 Ernst Cassirer, *Language and Myth*. Trans. Suzanne Langer. (New York: Dover, 1946). See pages 44-62.

4 Henri Bergson, *Le rire, essai sur la signification du comique* (Paris: Félix Alcan, 1913).

5 Forster, E.M., *Aspects of the Novel*. 1927; rpt. (San Diego: Harcourt Brace Jovanovich, 1985).

6 Steve Martin, "Artist Lost to Zoloft." In *Pure Drivel* (New York: Hyperion, 1998), 58-62.

7 Sigmund Freud, *Wit and Its Relation to the Unconscious*. Trans. James Strachey. (New York: W. W. Norton, 1960). Originally published as *Der Witze und seine Beziehung zum Unbewussen* in 1905.

Chapter Four

1 Genevieve Noone Parsons, Sara B. Kinsman, Charles L. Bosk, Pamela Sanka, and Peter A. Ubel, "Medical Student Perceptions of Humor and Slang in the Hospital Setting" *Journal of General Internal Medicine* 16 (2001): 544-549.

2 Posting of February 8, 2010; used by permission of Dr. Baruch.

3 T. Lagu, E. J. Kaufman, D. A. Asch, et al., "Content of Weblogs Written by Health Professionals." *Journal of General Internal Medicine* 23.10 (2008): 1642-1646. S. H. Jain, "Practicing Medicine in the Age of Facebook." *NEJM* 361 (2009): 649-651. K. C. Chretien et al., "Online Posting of Unprofessional Content by Medical Students," *JAMA* 302 (2009): 1309-1315.

4 Thich Nhat Hanh, *Being Peace* (Berkeley: Parallax Press, 1987), p. 5.

5 Lynne McTaggart, *The Intention Experiment: Using Your Thoughts to Change Your Life and the World* (New York: Free Press, 2007), p. xvii.

6 Wayne W. Dyer, *The Power of Intention: Learning to Co-create Your World Your Way* (Carlsbad, Calif.: Hay House, 2004).

7 Johan Huizinga, *Homo Ludens: A Study of the Play Element in Culture* (Boston: Beacon, 1950).

8 Delese Wear, Julie M. Aultman, Joseph D. Varley, and Joseph Zarconi. "Making Fun of Patients: Medical Students' Perceptions and Use of Derogatory and Cynical Humor in Clinical Settings," *Academic Medicine* 81.5 (2006): 454-462.

9 Albert Howard Carter, III, *First Cut: A Season in the Human Anatomy Lab* (New

York: Picador, 1997).

10 For various overviews, see Jim Holt, *Stop Me If You've Heard This: A History and Philosophy of Jokes* (New York: W. W. Norton, 2008), Ted Cohen, *Jokes: Philosophical Thoughts on Joking Matters* (Chicago: Univ. of Chicago Press, 1999), and John Allen Paulos, *I Think, Therefore I Laugh* (New York: Columbia Univ. Press, 2000). It's always interesting to see philosophy trying to make sense of jokes, when clearly there's a strong intuitive and emotional content in jokes and in our responses to them.

11 Madelijn Strick, Rob W. Holland, Rick B. van Baaren, Ad van Knippenberg, "Finding Comfort in a Joke: Consolatory Effects of Humor through Cognitive Distraction," *Emotion* 9.4 (2009): 574-578.

Chapter Five

1 Jonathan Culler, *On Puns: The Foundation of Letters* (Oxford: Basil Blackwell, 1988).

2 Mark Leyner and Billy Goldberg, M.D., *Let's Play Doctor: The Instant Guide to Walking, Talking, and Probing Like a Real M.D.* (New York: Crown, 2008).

3 A knight is on his quest when his faithful steed collapses and dies. The knight lugs his gear to the next town and visits the stable. The ostler shows him one horse after another, all not up to knightly standards: too large, too small, wrong color, wrong breed, wrong name, etc. [This process can be dragged out to any length.] In the last stall, there's a very large, robust, and handsome Saint Bernard, which smiles and wags its tail. The knight is very impressed and says he would like to purchase this fine beast and ride it onwards straightaway and forthwith.

The ostler, hat in hand, shakes his head and says, "Oh no, sir, I wouldn't send a knight out on a dog like this!"

4 Bernard J. Freedman, *Just a Word, Doctor: A Light-Hearted Guide to Medical Terms* (Oxford: Oxford Univ. Press, 1987).

Chapter Seven

1 John W. Draper, *The Humors & Shakespeare's Characters* (Durham: Duke Univ. Press, 1945).

2 *The New Yorker Book of Doctor Cartoons* (New York: Alfred A. Knopf, 1993).

3 Wendy Northcott, *The Darwin Awards 4: Intelligent Design* (New York: Dutton, 2006).

Chapter Eight

1 Sigmund Freud, *Jokes and Their Relation to the Unconscious*. Trans. James Strachey. New York: W. W. Norton, 1960. *The Interpretation of Dreams*. Trans. A. A. Brill. (New York: Macmillan, 1933).
2 Marc Galanter, *Lowering the Bar: Lawyer Jokes & Legal Culture* (Madison: University of Wisconsin Press, 2005).

Chapter Ten

1 Barron H. Lerner, "Future Doctors Behaving Badly: Dancing with Skeletons and Mocking Dermatologists in Medical-Student Comedy Shows," *Slate*, posted online Nov. 7, 2008.
2 Suzanne Poirier, *Doctors in the Making: Memoirs and Medical Education* (Iowa City: Univ. of Iowa Press, 2009).
3 Perri Klass, *Not an Entirely Benign Procedure* (New York: Putnam, 1987).

Chapter Twelve

1 Cecil B. DeMille's version in 1929 had Gary Cooper say, "When you call me that—smile." See http://www.answers.com/topic/the-virginian-1946-film, accessed January 28, 2010.
2 See Eric Weiner, *The Geography of Bliss* (New York: Twelve, 2008), p. 110.
3 Hunald Hasan and Tasneem Fatema Hasan, "Laugh Yourself into a Healthier Person: A Cross Cultural Analysis of the Effects of Varying Levels of Laughter on Health," *International Journal of Medical Sciences* 6(4) (2009): 200-211.
4 Kathryn Montgomery, *How Doctors Think: Clinical Judgment and the Practice of Medicine* (Oxford: Oxford Univ. Press, 2006) and Jerome Groopman, *How Doctors Think* (Boston: Houghton Mifflin, 2007).
5 K. N. Adamle, R. Ludwick, "Humor in Hospice Care: Who, Where, and How Much?" *American Journal of Hospice and Palliative Medicine* 22(4) (2005): 287-90.
6 Atul Gawande, *The Checklist Manifesto: How to Get Things Right* (New York: Henry Holt, 2010).

Bibliography

Adamle, K.N. and R. Ludwick. "Humor in Hospice Care: Who, Where, and How Much?" *American Journal of Hospice and Palliative Medicine* 22(4) (2005): 287-90.

Bachelard, Gaston. *The Poetics of Space.* Trans. Maria Jolas. Boston: Beacon, 1969.

Barber, Cesar Lombardy. *Shakespeare's Festive Comedy: A Study of Dramatic Form and Its Relation to Social Custom.* Princeton: Princeton Univ. Press, 1959.

Bauby, Jean-Dominique. *The Diving Bell and the Butterfly.* Trans. Jeremy Leggatt. New York: Knopf, 1997.

Bergson, Henri. *Le rire, essai sur la signification du comique.* Paris: Félix Alcan, 1913.

Campbell, Joseph. *The Hero with A Thousand Faces.* 1949; rpt. rev. ed. Princeton Univ. Press, 1968.

Carter, III, Albert Howard. *First Cut: A Season in the Human Anatomy Lab.* New York: Picador, 1997.

_____. "Literary Analogues to Living Wills." In *Advance Directives in Medicine.* Eds. Chris Hackler, Ray Mosley, and Dorothy E. Vawter. New York: Praeger, 1987: 181-87.

_____. *Our Human Hearts: A Medical and Cultural Journey.* Kent Ohio: Kent State Univ. Press, 2006.

_____ and Jane Arbuckle Petro. *Rising from the Flames: The Experience of the Severely Burned.* Philadelphia: Univ. of Pennsylvania Press, 1998.

Cassirer, Ernst. *Language and Myth.* Trans. Suzanne Langer. New York: Dover, 1946.

Cassell, Eric J. *The Healer's Art.* Cambridge: MIT Press, 1985.

Charon, Rita. *Narrative Medicine: Honoring the Stories of Illness.* Oxford, New York: Oxford Univ. Press, 2006.

Chretien, K. C., et al. "Online Posting of Unprofessional Content by Medical Students." *JAMA* 302 (2009): 1309-1315.

Cohen, Ted. *Jokes: Philosophical Thoughts on Joking Matters.* Chicago: Univ. of Chicago Press, 1999.

Culler, Jonathan. *On Puns: The Foundation of Letters.* Oxford: Basil Blackwell, 1988.

Draper, John W. *The Humors & Shakespeare's Characters*. Durham: Duke Univ. Press, 1945.

Dyer, Wayne W. *The Power of Intention: Learning to Co-create Your World Your Way*. Carlsbad, Calif.: Hay House, 2004.

Freedman, Bernard J. *Just a Word, Doctor: A Light-Hearted Guide to Medical Terms*. Oxford: Oxford Univ. Press, 1987.

Forster, E. M. *Aspects of the Novel*. 1927; rpt. San Diego: Harcourt Brace Jovanovich, 1985.

Freud, Sigmund. *Wit and Its Relation to the Unconscious*. Trans. James Strachey. New York: W. W. Norton, 1960. Originally published as *Der Witze und seine Beziehung zum Unbewussen* in 1905.

———. *The Interpretation of Dreams*. Trans. A. A. Brill. New York: Macmillan, 1933.

Frye, Northrop. *Anatomy of Criticism*. Princeton, Princeton Univ. Press, 1957.

Galanter, Marc. *Lowering the Bar: Lawyer Jokes & Legal Culture*. Madison: University of Wisconsin Press, 2005.

Gawande, Atul. *The Checklist Manifesto: How to Get Things Right*. New York: Henry Holt, 2010.

Groopman, Jerome. *How Doctors Think*. Boston: Houghton Mifflin, 2007.

Hanh, Thich Nhat. *Being Peace*. Berkeley: Parallax Press, 1987.

Hasan, Hunald, and Tasneem Fatema Hasan, "Laugh Yourself into a Healthier Person: A Cross Cultural Analysis of the Effects of Varying Levels of Laughter on Health." *International Journal of Medical Sciences* 6(4) (2009): 200-211.

Holt, Jim. *Stop Me If You've Heard This: A History and Philosophy of Jokes*. New York: W. W. Norton, 2008.

Huizinga, Johan. *Homo Ludens: A Study of the Play Element in Culture*. Boston: Beacon, 1950

Hunter, Kathryn Montgomery. *Doctors' Stories: The Narrative Structure of Medical Knowledge*. Princeton, NJ: Princeton Univ. Press, 1991.

Jain, S. H. "Practicing Medicine in the Age of Facebook." *NEJM* 361 (2009): 649-651.

Klass, Perri. *Not an Entirely Benign Procedure*. New York: Putnam, 1987.

Kruse, Barbara G., and Mark Prazak "Humor and Older Adults: What Makes them Laugh," *Journal of Holistic Nursing* 24 (2006): 188-193, 192.

Kübler-Ross, Elisabeth. *On Death and Dying*. New York: Macmillan, 1969.

Lagu,T., E. J. Kaufman, D. A. Asch, et al., "Content of Weblogs Written by Health Professionals." *Journal of General Internal Medicine* 23.10 (2008): 1642-1646.

Lerner, Barron H. "Future Doctors Behaving Badly: Dancing with Skeletons and

Mocking Dermatologists in Medical-Student Comedy Shows." *Slate*, posted online Nov. 7, 2008.

Leyner, Mark, and Billy Goldberg, M.D., *Let's Play Doctor: The Instant Guide to Walking, Talking, and Probing Like a Real M.D.* New York: Crown, 2008.

McMahan, Selena Clare. "Infinite Possibility: Clowning with Elderly People." *Care Management Journals* 9.1 (2008): 19-24.

McTaggart, Lynne. *The Intention Experiment: Using Your Thoughts to Change Your Life and the World.* New York: Free Press, 2007.

Martin, Steve "Artist Lost to Zoloft." In *Pure Drivel.* New York: Hyperion, 1998, 58-62.

Maxwell, W. "The Use of Gallows Humor and Dark Humor During Crisis Situations." *International Journal of Emergency Mental Health* 5.2 (2003): 93-98.

Montgomery, Kathryn. *How Doctors Think: Clinical Judgment and the Practice of Medicine.* Oxford, New York: Oxford Univ. Press, 2006.

The New Yorker Book of Doctor Cartoons. New York: Alfred A. Knopf, 1993.

Northcott, Wendy. *The Darwin Awards 4: Intelligent Design.* New York: Dutton, 2006.

Parsons, Genevieve Noone, Sara B. Kinsman, Charles L. Bosk, Pamela Sanka, and Peter A. Ubel. "Medical Student Perceptions of Humor and Slang in the Hospital Setting." *Journal of General Internal Medicine* 16 (2001): 544-549.

Paulos, John Allen. *I Think, Therefore I Laugh.* New York: Columbia Univ. Press, 2000.

Poirier, Suzanne. *Doctors in the Making: Memoirs and Medical Education.* Iowa City: Univ. of Iowa Press, 2009.

Solzhenitsyn, Alexander. *Cancer Ward.* Translated by Nicholas Bethell and David Burg. New York: Modern Library, 1983.

Sontag, Susan. *Illness as Metaphor and AIDS and Its Metaphors.* New York: Picador, 1989.

Strick, Madelijn, Rob W. Holland, Rick B. van Baaren, and Ad van Knippenberg. "Finding Comfort in a Joke: Consolatory Effects of Humor through Cognitive Distraction." *Emotion* 9.4 (2009): 574-578.

Vagnoli, L., S. Caprilli, A. Robiglio, and A. Messeri, "Clown Doctors as a Treatment for Preoperative Anxiety in Children: A Randomized, Prospective Study." *Pediatrics* 116.4 (2005): 563-7.

Wald, Barbara, et al. "Clowns in der Psychiatrie? Ein Pilotprojekt." *Nervenarzt* 78.5 (June 2007): 571-74.

Wear, Delese, Julie M. Aultman, Joseph D. Varley, and Joseph Zarconi. "Making Fun of Patients: Medical Students' Perceptions and Use of Derogatory and Cynical

Humor in Clinical Settings." *Academic Medicine* 81.5 (2006): 454-462.

Weiner, Eric. *The Geography of Bliss.* New York: Twelve, 2008.

Wilson, Edward O. *Biophilia.* Cambridge, Mass.: Harvard Univ. Press, 1984.

Woodruff, Lee, and Bob Woodruff. *In an Instant: A Family's Journey of Love and Healing.* New York: Random House, 2007.

Index

K